SUMMER OF SEXINESS:
A Self Awakening

A Memoir by Jeannie X

Prologue

To a certain extent, I am not really sure where to begin because in some ways this story starts in May 2018; in others, it begins a few years before that; but, if I am really honest, it has its origins in my early 20s, when I was first out of college. Back then, I was enjoying being single, launching my career and trying to figure out what I wanted from my life. And, what I wanted from my sex life.

I dated around at first and then proceeded to fall in and out of love with a number of different men, each one bringing his own unique set of characteristics that captivated me at the time. For the most part, I felt comfortable having sex with these men.

Eventually, I decided to pursue a long-term relationship with the man, Viktor, who became my husband, but even though we initially had a lot of sexual chemistry, it disappeared soon after I moved in with him.

I had been sexually active in college and, as a single woman in New York City, thought that I was a well-adjusted, sexually empowered woman. Yet, I was wrong. Instead, I was sexually shut down, filled with immense shame and lacking in sexual desire and libido. It turned out that I was less well-adjusted in general as well.

At first, I attributed my lack of desire to depression, having just uprooted myself from one state to another to be with Viktor. Then, I blamed birth control pills. But, despite making changes to address these supposed causes, nothing changed. And I felt so at odds with being a wife and being a sexual being (perhaps it was too many episodes of *Donna Reed?*).

By then, I was convinced that I was "broken" and turned to traditional therapy to "fix" me. Yet, even with years spent talking to one therapist after another, I was still without any sustained interest in sex. For over a decade, I lived in a loving, yet nearly sexless, marriage. We were physically affectionate, but if we had intercourse more than once a month, it was a lot.

Thankfully, my husband was patient and loving, choosing me without sex, rather than leaving me for someone else. But I knew I wanted more...so much more. This was not what I had wanted for myself or for our partnership, but I felt stuck, shut down and stifled. I didn't give up hope, but I was at a loss as to how to make any actual progress.

In 2006, I had my answer in the form of a newly opened pole dance studio called S Factor. Since that first class, my S journey has been a vital part of my sexual exploration as I learned to truly take ownership of my sexuality and sensuality, at least within the confines of the studio. It was an important first step.

A few years later, I enrolled in Mama Gena's School of the Womanly Arts' Mastery Program. I knew that this was the next piece of the puzzle and through my work with Regena Thomashauer (aka Mama Gena) and my immersion in her Sister Goddess community, I started to plant seeds, overcoming body shame and finally stepping into my sexual power.

Throughout this journey, my husband has been my steadfast supporter, lover, and confidante. I have never once doubted that we were meant to be together or wavered in my love for him. We have spent countless hours talking about our sex life (or lack thereof), experienced numerous failed attempts to infuse more sex into our lives and discovered many wins along the way as we studied with sexologist Miss Jaiya, participated in Tantra classes, and explored the D/s world.

And, for over four years we had incredible discussions about threesomes, open marriages, and polyamory. In the beginning, I was hesitant to bring it up, but I felt that it was something that I had to give voice to. Yes, that first conversation was scary, but then, once it was over, I noticed something remarkably interesting. Our talk about bringing in other partners was actually pulling us closer together rather than pushing us apart, as we bared our souls and got intimate in the most vulnerable and honest of ways.

Concurrently, while I was intrigued by these conversations, I was also terrified that such a move on either of our parts would potentially damage the beautiful foundation we had built over our two decades of marriage. We continued to verbally explore these ideas; sharing what elements were tantalizing, which weren't and what we ultimately wanted from such an arrangement. Each time we talked, our foundation grew more solid and I knew that it would be strong enough to hold us in this next chapter of our journey.

Which brings us back to May 2018 when I attended an erotic party. Admittedly, I had no idea what to expect and was extremely nervous before I arrived, but thanks to the support of a dear friend, we ventured into the unknown together, kicking off what became a wild ride.

So, what happens when a happily married couple explores the world of open relationships? Read on. This is my story of how I overcame sexual shutdown and shame and stepped into my true unapologetic self!

Part One

A first time for everything

Some people wait until they are married to have sex for the first time. Others lose their virginity in the heat of the moment...perhaps in the back seat of a car. For me, it was somewhere in between.

It was 1989; I was 18, a college freshman and very much in love with my college boyfriend, Ian, an upperclassman. We had met early in the fall semester and by the spring, we were in a committed, monogamous relationship, regularly spending weekends together in his room at the fraternity house.

Initially, we were kissing and petting, but not much more was happening. I had limited dating experience in high school. In fact, all throughout high school, I had been a bit boy crazy, desperately wanting a boyfriend, but was never asked out.

Rather, in freshman year of high school, through a weird conflation of events, I found myself alone with a cute guy in his parents' house. We went into his room, laid down on the bed and started to kiss. Things progressed quickly from there. He first put his hand under my shirt and easily opened my front-hook bra, man-handling my breasts once he did so. I lay there motionless, feeling fear, not desire.

He then tried to go further, but, thankfully, I was wearing side-zip (as opposed to front zip) jeans and he wasn't able to figure out where the zipper was to remove my pants. I didn't know how to say "No," so I simply lay there hoping he would stop soon. I think I eventually extricated myself from his grip, noting that I needed to go home to do my homework.

I foolishly thought we would start dating, but he had simply used me and a few weeks later, at the start of the Jewish holiday of Yom Kippur (Day of Atonement), I found myself bawling loudly in synagogue feeling intense shame for having engaged in such sexual behavior.

Beyond that traumatic experience, there were just some occasional first dates and a hook-up on a family vacation my senior year, where I had given a handjob to a guy I had met. So, sex (especially intercourse) was foreign and a bit scary.

My mother had been a virgin on her wedding night and, while my parents were very forthcoming about the birds and the bees, taking me to the American Museum of Natural History's human sexuality exhibit, the message they gave me was clear: wait to have sex until I had a wedding ring on my finger. And the focus of their sexual education was on the mechanics of how things worked and where babies came from; not once did they mention pleasure or orgasms.

Moreover, growing up amidst the AIDS epidemic, the fear of death from sex was real. I remember talking with a friend who was about to go off to college when I was still in high school about how we had been cheated. All of the sexual gains that had been made during the 1960s and 1970s were no longer available to us; sex could kill. While not yet ready to engage in sex myself, I keenly felt the loss that our opportunity to be fully sexually free had been taken away from us.

With all of this in mind, I felt strongly about connecting with my college boyfriend in a more intimate way and Ian and I began to talk about having sex. I don't remember all of those conversations, but I do know that I was willing, but very anxious. He let on that he had some experience with a previous partner and I eventually decided that I was ready to take this next step.

At the time, sex was initially all about love. At least that was what I had assimilated from my parents. In preparation for this momentous moment, I asked my mother to make an appointment with her gynecologist so I could go on the birth control pill. While she openly wished I would wait for marriage, she agreed to be supportive, made the appointment and took me to the doctor's office when I was home for Spring Break. In addition to the medical visit, she took me to purchase a dainty negligee for the occasion, wanting to be sure the night was romantic and special.

Despite my bravado at planning ahead, admittedly, I was extremely nervous. While I had earned top grades in health class and seen the exhibit at the museum, I still didn't understand how Tab A was magically supposed to fit into Slot B. I mean, logically I understood it, but it seemed like it would be much more complicated in reality.

On the night in question, Ian and I went to dinner and then returned to his room, lit some candles, put on music and began to kiss. I continued to be nervous but tried to relax. I knew my body so little at the time and can't recall if I had even had an orgasm by then. Probably not.

After a while we proceeded to have intercourse. Of course, it was awkward and painful, but we figured it out. It turned out that Ian had lied to comfort me and was a virgin, too. I was equally upset that he had deceived me and secretly pleased that I was also his first. Afterwards, I felt a mix of emotions. I was somewhat confused by what all the fuss and hype was about. Why were people breaking rules, jeopardizing marriages and otherwise risking their life? I didn't feel any magical moment. However, I was incredibly happy to have connected so deeply with my guy. I commemorated the occasion in my diary at the time:

"Last night Ian and I made love for the first time. It was so beautiful. I love him with all my heart...I hope it continues to get better because it's still a little painful and it's not as fantastic feeling-wise as I thought it would be. It was great because I loved being so intimate with Ian, but it didn't seem to be such a fabulous thing like everyone says it is...I don't know, there doesn't seem to be much to do except rotate your pelvis/hips. Well, next week we'll be at it again. God, I love him."

(And, a year later, I left myself an editor's note: "The above sounds childish and stupid, it embarrasses me."

Ian and I continued to have sex throughout our relationship, which lasted for another year. Interestingly, neither of us was particularly creative nor inventive, so we basically stuck with missionary position each time (at least that's the way I remember it). And my pleasure was less important...to both of us. In fact, it wasn't until I was visiting him during the following Spring Break that we took a shower together and he went down on me for the first time. Wow! I was finally feeling something intense, but I don't think I climaxed with him then or ever.

Ian and I essentially broke up at the end of my sophomore year since he had graduated from college and moved to Orlando, Florida. I would visit him on occasion, but we both agreed to date other people.

But, in spite of my carefully curated loss of virginity, I didn't fully own my sexuality, instead I gave it away to men in exchange for attention and permitted men to take even when I wasn't into it.

That autumn, I returned to school, ready to start my junior year and excited about what was to come. I had a great off-campus apartment with some friends, held a leadership position with my sorority and was active with several other extracurricular activities including the student newspaper, an organization with which I had participated the year before. During that time, I had met Robert and immediately developed a crush on him. We would run into each other at various events on campus and I would flirt with him. I wanted him to ask me out and at some point, I gave him my phone number.

A few weeks into the semester, he finally called...at 2:00 a.m. He invited me to come to his apartment and I naively went, thinking that he actually liked me and wanted to start dating. Upon arrival, we headed to his room and began to make out. I was flattered that he was interested in me and was excited to potentially have a new boyfriend. Things escalated from kissing quite quickly and soon, I was in just my bra and panties, then only a little while later, I was fully naked.

I wasn't sure what was happening since I still had such limited experience. Soon we were having sexual intercourse, even though I didn't really want to. I didn't have the words or the confidence to say no. I simply did what I thought he wanted as a way to get him to ask me out. I stupidly thought he genuinely returned my feelings and that this was the start of something, not a beginning, middle and end all in one night.

But the truth of the situation became crystal clear and by the next night, I was an emotional wreck. The shame and negative feelings hit me hard and were overwhelming. I was disgusted with myself and felt angry and defiled. It wasn't quite rape because I never said no, but I really didn't want to be having sex with him. I felt as though I had lost my innocence, writing in my journal that I would "never be the same person I was. I feel slutty, defiled and cheap. I didn't really enjoy it — I just went through the motions and there was no emotion behind it."

Over the next few months, I turned the blame inward and fell into a deep depression, all the while trying to justify what had happened. In an attempt to normalize the situation, I invited him to dinner one night and we had sex again, creating a false sense of a relationship to make myself feel better about having had sex with him the first time. I was just fooling myself, but I didn't know how else to handle the intense shame and self-hatred. By December, I nearly took my own life in a (thankfully) failed suicide attempt.

I found myself in a scared, fearful place, afraid to date, in recognition that men were so hung up on sex. I knew that I didn't want to be touched sexually. I kept remembering what had happened with Robert believing that my worst men fears were confirmed. I couldn't bear the thought of anything but hugs and maybe kisses. Anything else frightened me because it was too possible to lead beyond and then become inevitable for sex to occur.

Moreover, I still felt guilty and defiled for what had happened with Robert since I believed (in hindsight) that I could have said no and simply left but instead had let it happen and didn't even protest. In retrospect, I could recognize that there was no threat, but am not so sure that's what I felt in the moment. At the same time, he played on my insecurities and desire for affection. I wondered if I would ever come to terms with that night noting that it lay in that obscure territory between consent and rape. I knew I needed help and time to heal.

Although the depression was primarily brought on by the sexual shame, there were other issues going on in my life, so I took the following semester off to nurse myself back to health. I saw a therapist, went on antidepressants, and began to reassess my life goals.

Life begins again

That summer, a friend and I rented a room in Manhattan for a month, which was an amazing time for me. Shortly before our lease began, my friend had found a boyfriend and thus spent lots of time with him. Eager to take advantage of living in the city (as opposed to my parents' house in the suburbs), I headed out every night whether it was to go to the movies, see a comedy show or simply sit in a coffee shop. I found courage and strength to do things on my own and by the fall, I was ready to go back to school.

Concurrent with living in the city, I was working at a law firm, where I had been employed the previous summer and then again, since my departure from school in January. I soon developed a big crush on my colleague Greg. I was attracted to his good looks and confidence but didn't expect anything to come of it.

One Friday afternoon at work, several of us were hanging out in the back office talking about sex and a dozen other topics. We were all being very silly and flirty with one another and I wrote on Greg's back with my finger, "You are very good looking" and "You are sexy." His fingers replied, "So are you." Swoon! Through a weird confluence of events, I ended up going back to his apartment that night, with the intention of simply hanging out and staying over (I had been supposed to meet up with someone else and stay over, but that date was cancelled.)

At that point, I hadn't really dated anyone (and certainly hadn't had sex with anyone) since Robert. Of course, between the fact that Greg was a sexy, 20-something man and my big crush on him, we ended up doing more than just hang out.

Initially Greg and I went back to his apartment, talked, watched television and drank a bit. I was having a wonderful time and we began to kiss. Afterwards, Greg and I went to his bedroom and began to fool around. At one point I found the courage to say, "I will sleep with you if you wear a condom." Not surprisingly, he immediately got dressed and headed to the nearest drug store, returning as quickly as possible.

I felt immensely powerful and in control in telling him what I wanted, ensuring that he adhered to my rules and in simply being desired. It was such a different experience from the one with Robert. I knew that Greg was experienced with women and had hoped for a more pleasurable sexual experience. It didn't quite happen that way, but I was so proud of myself, reclaiming my sexual self after the pain and shame of Robert.

Greg told me I was cute and sexy and very attractive and that I could use all of it to my advantage. He also said I had a great body. His compliments and attention were definitely a confidence booster and I knew he was sincere. He had given me so much in one night than he would ever know. As I wrote the next day, "My life begins again today. I no longer fear sex or men."

A few months later, I put this lesson to the test. I was sitting at my desk at work and answered a call for Greg. It was his friend Ben. When I gave Greg the phone message, I jokingly asked if Ben had a girlfriend and Greg offered to set me up with him.

After some missed calls and connections, Ben and I eventually had our first date, which went rather well. I happily accepted a second date during which we talked and talked and didn't seem to run out of anything to say. Among the varied topics, he asked me if I had a summer home in which I could "squirrel him away, cook for him and give him a massage." I replied that while I didn't have a summer home, I did have an apartment in Ithaca (I still had my off-campus apartment). He thought that was a great idea and we picked a mutually convenient weekend to head upstate.

As he stood with me waiting for a cab to take me home, he promised to return the favor of a massage and said that he had taken lessons on the weekends during his undergraduate days at Brown. He even used his own oils. I was intrigued, but also a little wary since oils seemed to imply bare backs and bare backs implied nudity to me. I thought that I might like to sleep with him, but not for a long time...not until I was sure that I was in love and that he felt almost, if not the same, way.

I eagerly anticipated our weekend away, looking forward to showing him around campus and having two days of uninterrupted time to get to know each other. But I was also nervous. I wasn't ready to sleep with him and wasn't tempted to "cheat" and give in before I was ready. I trusted myself to wait until the love between us was truly there.

Once up at school, Ben and I had a fun time together, although I did turn down his request to sleep with him. On Sunday morning, we lay in bed talking and then kissing. Things began to escalate as he touched my breasts and caressed my body. He eventually found his way between my legs and under my panties, noticing the moisture and then vocalizing, "You are so wet." I was mortified and felt shame wash over me. Yes, I knew that lubrication was normal and natural, but to have it so distinctly pointed out was too much for me to handle.

We headed home and he called the next day to say that things were over (not that they really ever began), but still, it stung, and I was certain that the lack of sex was a big part of his motivation to break up. But I was also pleased that I had remained truthful to myself and what I did — and didn't — want sexually from him.

I returned to campus in the fall, in a good mood, and feeling ready to face the world again. It was my senior year and I turned 21. That fall entailed a collection of crushes and occasional dates. It was a fun diversion as I settled back into school after my semester and summer off. There were the usual ups and downs, but then things faded as quickly as they began. I dated sporadically and attracted the attention of a few guys, but nothing serious developed. I fooled around with some of them, but I didn't have sex with anyone.

That spring semester included an on-again, off-again relationship with Brian, who wanted a commitment, while I only wanted to have fun. In the process, I hooked up with my friend Mike, invited him to my formal, disinvited Brian, etc. Typical college drama.

At the end of the spring term, I was excited for graduation and senior week. I would still have another semester of classes in the fall to make up for the one I had missed, but I was eager to celebrate with my friends. By the time classes had ended and Senior Week arrived, I felt free to do what I wanted, when I wanted and with whom I wanted. And, of course, I exploited this to the fullest that week.

During senior week, I found my sexual power, flirting with various men and ended up having several one-night stands. It became a fun game that infused me with confidence.

I kicked off the week flirting shamelessly with one guy after another on our winery tour and then again that night while out at various bars with friends. After leaving the bars that first night, I was standing on the street with my friend Marie, who introduced me to Jeff. Jeff and I talked for a bit and then proceeded to dance right in the middle of town as he spun and dipped me, which was fun. Soon Marie had conveniently disappeared, and Jeff took me home with him. I spent the night and we fooled around but didn't have sex. I might have if he had asked, but he never asked. I was simply happy that he hadn't used that horrible line, "I want to be inside you," which (at the time) I found to be gross.

The next night, I recognized this guy Adam, considered him to be a challenge and set out to see what I could accomplish. I tentatively approached him and was met with a friendly demeanor. Adam and I hung out with his friends, as I flirted with him. A lot. As the bar closed, Adam initially indicated an interest in going to an after party, but he then changed his mind and began to kiss me. I knew that I had succeeded in my quest. He took me home with him.

Back at his apartment, Adam took me to his room. We fooled around for a while, slowly undressing, until we were almost nude. Adam asked me if I wanted to make love. I thought it was a rather poor choice of words — it's sex, I didn't love him — but at least he asked and didn't use that "inside you" line. He was fun and I spent the night. The next morning, I reflected on the fun experience and wondered what other mischief I could get myself into in the days remaining before graduation.

Thursday night included flirtations with Toby and Wesley, the latter of whom I had met freshman year and had a crush on. Upon this reunion (I hadn't seen Wesley since we were freshman), I reminded him about an episode in which he had been going off to play poker after a party we'd both attended, and I told him that I was more fun than poker. Unfortunately, he had gone off to the game. He said he remembered that night and that he'd always regretted going to play poker. After hanging out for several hours, Wesley invited me to his apartment where we fooled around a bit — mostly just kissing and then I slept there for the night.

Friday night, I resumed my flirtations with Toby, who was an aspiring photographer. Since I had never seen his portfolio, he brought me to his home to show it to me. His work was really good; mostly pictures from cafes from when he was in France for the semester. After two hours of talking, he finally kissed me. We proceeded to fool around heavily and then we were both nude. I asked him if he had a condom, but after a brief search, he didn't, so we obviously didn't have sex. By that time, it was 6:00 a.m., so I stayed the rest of night, sleeping for a few scant hours.

The final night of the celebrations found me hanging out with Oliver, who had been buying me beers earlier in the week. Later in the night, Oliver leaned over and asked if he could kiss me. I said yes and he responded accordingly. It felt a little weird to be kissing in a public place even though it was semi-dark. Then he asked me if I wanted to go back to his apartment with him. I thought about it for a moment and decided yes but advised him that I could only stay for a few hours since my parents were visiting for graduation.

Back at his apartment, we fooled around and then he said he wanted to make love to me. I asked if he had a condom, recalling the previous night's escapade. He said yes and we had sex. He was pretty good. We fooled around some more and then I said that I had to go even though I didn't want to.

Despite the transient nature of these hook-ups, instead of feeling tawdry as I had with Robert, I felt powerful and desired. I felt that I had wanted these encounters, actively pursued them and achieved my quarry. It was such a different feeling than that of feeling used and discarded. There was no shame, only success. Yet, it was still lacking in true desire and pleasure; there was no focus on my orgasm, only on those of the men. This was a missing piece of the puzzle, but I didn't perceive it at the time.

That summer found me dating a few men, including Wesley and Oliver from Senior Week. I had wondered if Oliver would call, since he had promised to do so. I mused as to whether he might think less of me because I slept with him without really knowing him but knew I wasn't (and didn't feel like) a slut. I knew that I had been clearly in control in all of these situations and knew I could say no to anything I didn't want to do. I enjoyed the power. Similarly, I pondered the ability to continue this behavior in the fall when it wasn't Senior Week and knew that I wouldn't be nearly so bold or reckless in the city, compared to the safety of campus.

On our date, Oliver took me to dinner and then we had a few beers at a bar in the West Village. We returned to my parents' apartment (they were away) and hung out, talking briefly, before we proceeded to have sex. We had sex twice during the night and then he left around 2:00 a.m. We got to know each other much better this time around, but I wasn't sure how I felt about him long term. He was very well-endowed, and it hurt to be with him physically. Despite my newfound power, I felt stupid to say anything, so I kept quiet and knew that it was my own fault that I was in pain after he left.

Conversely, things proceeded more slowly with Wesley, whose company I very much enjoyed, but I didn't get excited or turned on by him. I kept hoping that would change as I got to know him better but thought intuitively that if there weren't sparks from day one, there likely would never be sparks.

During this time, I referred to myself as "too sexual of a person" in a journal entry and further noted that, "It's only recently that people (men) have been complimenting me with the term sexy, but I know they see 'cute' much more than 'sexy.' But only I knew the truth."

By July, I was beginning to feel restless, noting a recurring feeling during this time of the year. I felt a lot of sexual tension building up, wanting desperately to be released, referring to myself as a sexual person who will not and cannot be labeled. I emphatically noted that, "I will do what I want with whom I want; I do not fit neatly into any category in any area of my life."

Yet at the same time, as I further reflected on Senior Week and the summer, I found myself thinking hard about the decisions I had made for myself and my lifestyle. In my journal, I characterized my behavior as "almost promiscuous" when it came to my hooking up, but now, although I had no regrets, I felt that such a lifestyle wasn't me. I also realized that I didn't need to be a prude either.

Rather, I just had to approach each situation uniquely, while valuing my own needs. I downplayed my sexual desire, noting that I wanted to get to know people better before I jumped into bed with them. I also wanted to make safety a number one priority, stating, "My life is much too important to sacrifice for a night of passion. I will not throw my life away." I was in a good place, acknowledging that I was growing stronger again, rebuilding my self-esteem and becoming the adult woman I was meant to be.

Will she or won't she?

But, clearly, there was some regret and shame lingering underneath. In August, I had just finished reading an enjoyable book, *Emma Who Saved My Life,*[1] that I had purchased at the Dollar Store, in which one of the characters chose to be celibate for over 10 years. I began to think that maybe this was a way to get to the truth of my sexuality. Perhaps celibacy could help me concentrate on other issues such as how sexual of a person I was. Was I able to remain celibate or not, keeping out of one-night stands and seeing who still stays around, and of course, avoiding venereal disease, AIDS, and pregnancy?

It seemed like a good idea and, when I resumed classes, I continued to mull over my proposed celibacy and told a few friends about the idea. The more I spoke about it, the better the idea seemed. I thought that a six-month trial basis would be a good start. Among the rules, I decided that kissing would be allowed, but nothing else could happen. Masturbation was also off-limits.

I admonished myself to be consistent, noting that I couldn't make exceptions for anyone. I told myself that this was a choice I was making for myself so that I could learn the truth about my sexuality. Was I as sexual a person as I had claimed to be and if so, to what extent? Did I want only sex or love or both? What did I want from my sexual life? I felt sure that the answers to all of these questions would only come with time.

I was confident that refraining from sexual encounters would permit me to be more in touch with my true feelings on this issue and knew that I would be greatly disappointed in myself if I was unable to make it through the trial period. Of course, this meant that the next time I had sex — six months from then — I would have a lot of choices to make. Would I want a one-night stand to end my celibacy or should I wait for a real relationship to develop?

---

[1] Barnhardt, Wilton. *Emma Who Saved My Life.* New York: Picador, 1989.

Two weeks into the experiment, I made the mistake of fantasizing in my head in an attempt to ward off insomnia. I allowed myself to imagine sexual encounters and let my imagination run wild. Before I knew it, I was very excited and very stimulated. It got to a point where I decided that I needed to release the tension, so I allowed myself to manually finish what I had started. I was surprised at how far I had gotten with just my thoughts.

While I was dismayed with myself for getting into the situation, I realized that I could use this information. If I could learn to concentrate the way I did that night, I could get myself aroused much more quickly and strongly for when I was with some guy, with the hope that maybe I'd achieve orgasm more readily. I knew that it was said that most of sex was in the mind anyway. But I don't think I really internalized this lesson at the time.

By November, I had made it three months without sex. I was glad that I had succeeded, noting that I had learned a lot. I believed that I was, indeed, a sexual person, but not one controlled by her sexual feelings. I hadn't even kissed a boy in two months. I continued to be a big flirt but planned to remain celibate until the right relationship came along.

I began to feel that I had given my body away for the sake of sex and, instead, wanted to make love again. I wanted to be loved. I thought that this celibacy period had given me back a better perspective on sex. But had it? I felt the need to respect myself more, which was, of course, a good thing. Yet, I was denying myself pleasure. On one occasion, I almost hooked up when I got lonely and very drunk, but sent him home before anything really happened, when I started to feel nauseous.

In the morning I was extremely relieved that all that had transpired was five minutes of drunken kissing. I told myself that I wanted a relationship before I fooled around with someone. While I don't doubt that it was in my best interest to avoid having sex with a random stranger, in my naivety, I was unaware of what I was doing to myself. It was only decades later when I shared this celibacy experiment with a therapist that I recognized the hurt, pain and shame I was inflicting on myself.

I eventually finished up my final semester, officially graduated and moved home with my parents who had graciously had the foresight to sell their suburban home and move to Manhattan. I was living the life I had dreamed of — working in an office, hanging out with friends on the weekends and generally enjoying myself.

I was also enjoying the dating scene and had fun meeting men and feeling sexy and desired. After years of feeling like the ugly duckling, this was still new to me. I didn't expect to get married at a young age and was happy being single. I only dated men but did fantasize about dating a woman; I just didn't know how to go about it without making the person feel like a science experiment, so I never pursued it.

My first on-going boyfriend during that time was Wesley. We had started dating during the summer and then resumed things once I had graduated. We spent nearly every weekend together, going out either Friday or Saturday and then I would return home on Sunday night. We were sexually active, and our relationship included my first encounter with erectile dysfunction.

One night when I was with Wesley, we were really getting to know each other. Then we began fooling around. At first it was just kissing, then it rapidly progressed until we were both nude. Once Wesley put on a condom, things became somewhat difficult. Wesley's cock wasn't hard enough to engage in sexual intercourse.

After a few minutes of trying, it became apparent that we weren't going to have sex. I assumed that it was a rare thing for him, but it was a new experience for me. I was aware that such moments could be very embarrassing for men and I wanted to make sure that I was caring and supportive. I wasn't sure what to do. I didn't want to vocalize the situation for fear that it might make him feel worse.

Instead, I told him that I had a better idea. I removed the condom and decided that I would get him off with a blowjob. I kissed him and made my way down towards his penis. I wanted to take my time, but he wasn't responding at all. I was definitely confused. It wasn't something I was used to and wasn't prepared to know how to deal with the problem. So, I went a step further and placed his penis in my mouth. He finally got an erection and, after only a few minutes in my mouth, he came.

I knew that I shouldn't draw too much attention to his impotence, but I did want to better understand what was happening. He advised me that I intimidated him. What did that mean? I don't think I ever really knew. Moreover, how could a 4'-10" woman be so intimidating to a grown man?

Wesley and I continued to date, but I wasn't sure where things were headed. I didn't want to become friends with benefits. I either wanted an actual relationship or to remain strictly platonic. I was still marking time with my celibacy due to Wesley's issues, getting to the five month and eventually the six-month mark, officially completing my quest.

In the meantime, I had relaxed my other restrictions in the context of our relationship. One morning, after the alarm had gone off, Wesley and I held each other and kissed and then let things escalate. Wesley was more adventurous in the morning than he had been previously and began to rub my clitoris in an attempt to bring me to orgasm. Or rather, he tried; his finger was a little above where he needed to be, and I never really got going but I kind of pretended I did just to gracefully end his labors.

Later, I reflected on the fact that I hadn't felt comfortable to guide his hand or voice any direction so again, I knew it was my own fault. Moreover, to reward his efforts I gave him a blowjob. In spite of my quest for truth as a sexual being, I was still putting others' needs ahead of mine and blaming myself for my sexual shortcomings. I was not fully comfortable to speak up or ask for what I wanted. But I was blind to these issues at the time.

After several attempts at intercourse over several months, Wesley and I finally had penetrative sex after seven months of my celibacy. It was still a challenge for him to keep his erection, but with persistence, we made love for the first time. But it wasn't actually love. Yes, I was in love with him, but he didn't return the feelings.

Around this time, I met a guy named Doug to whom I was very sexually attracted. We went to a dance club and had an amazing time. There was something about him that was so provocative I could feel even when we were just talking. We were talking about sex and from what he was saying I decided right then that I wanted to sleep with him. We would dance for a long time, get really sweaty and then take a break. We would basically lean against a wall on each other and be very flirtatious and talk and kiss. It was great.

I told him that I found him incredibly sexy and he told me that he thought that I was sexy too. It was so cool to be with him and have him think of me as sexy, which was one of the compliments I had always strived for. Part of it was that Doug made me feel sexy. Around 2:00 a.m. we decided to leave the club and returned to my apartment. We fooled around quite intensely with all of this passion and lust behind it, but only above the waist.

In the wake of this experience, I now realized that after being celibate for seven months I was back to being a sexual person. Part of it was the fun, part of it was the attention that it brought me. I didn't need a relationship or emotion to have sex with someone, that wasn't what sex was to me. However, that didn't mean that I was going to go out and sleep with every man that winked at me. I reflected that I preferred a fun relationship with sex to a one-night stand, but the point was that I was in control and I made the decisions.

I felt excited about the new insight and that I finally understood myself and my sexual nature. I was coming to the truth of the matter and this was particularly important. Therefore, I felt that my experiment had worked in that regard. But it definitely had not been fun; it was simply a learning experience.

I continued to date Doug and eventually we had sex. He was absolutely as sexy as I had thought he would be, but for some reason I wasn't as turned on as I had been the week before. I found him to be relatively talented and quite different from Wesley; he was much more assertive and active.

Simultaneously, I was still seeing Wesley, but things weren't as rosy as they had been. I wasn't sure that he found me attractive or sexy. And, while I believed that "the sex between us is great" (whatever I meant by that in my journal), I was always the initiator and he never seemed as eager as I expected him to be. I wanted to explore more sexually with Wesley. I came to realize that I was a much more sexual person than he was — at least in that context — and it felt uncomfortable to remain in that situation. Not long after, we broke up.

Around this time, I discovered the writings of Anais Nin. I read her biography and saw so much of myself in her that it was eerie. It renewed my interest in a passionate, sexually liberating relationship. I felt that I needed attention from men as a stimulus of power and confidence. I wanted to flirt shamelessly then dash their hopes unless I really liked them. I wanted the dominance and control of the situation. Yet, I feared rejection and would seek out only those with whom I feel safe to pursue.

After the demise of my relationship with Wesley, other relationships followed, including those with Stanley, Kyle, Warren and Peter. Stanley and I had sex only a handful of times and it was more out of a sense of what I was supposed to do — what was expected — than what I really wanted. Interestingly, it was me that pushed the agenda, offering myself up to him on one of our dates, "I want you inside me." It was still all about intimate, emotional connection; the dots of pleasure were not yet connected.

Kyle and I had intense sexual chemistry, but he remained chaste due to his religious beliefs. Warren and I were more sexually adventurous, playing around with positions and locations. It was all fun and games, but it, too, came to an end. Peter and I had a brief relationship, fraught with miscommunication and only periodic sexual liaisons, again out of some sense of duty on my part. I suggested sex on New Year's Eve as we toasted the arrival of midnight and the coming year. It was perfunctory at best. Yet, there had also been love and connection.

Happily ever after?

A few months later, my then best friend and I went on vacation to Florida in February, where I had the wonderful opportunity to see my high school friend, Viktor. It had been nearly three years since we had seen each other in person, but we had always had an interest in one another beyond mere friendship.

Viktor and I had met in architecture class in high school when I was a senior and he was a junior. Soon after meeting him, I developed a strong crush on him, but he had a girlfriend and, while I joked to my friends about seducing him by candlelight, I never followed through on my plans. Instead, we became close friends, turning to one another throughout our college years.

Eventually, I disclosed my feelings for him, which he returned, but, with each of us in different parts of the country (me in upstate New York and him in New Orleans) and still in our late teens/early twenties, it wasn't something I wanted to pursue.

But there was definitely something growing between us. We became each other's confidante, sharing hopes, dreams and disappointments. Ours was a mutual meeting of hearts and minds and somehow, we could never be separated regardless of time and space. I constantly turned to him for guidance and he leaned on me for support. We would reconnect in person over holidays and school breaks, occasionally fooling around, but never letting it escalate too far. In fact, it wasn't until I had visited Florida on a previous trip that we finally decided to become more intimate.

I had been in Orlando visiting with Ian, my ex-boyfriend from college and then met up with Viktor who was living in Gainesville, Florida at the time. We had a lovely night out and I then returned to Viktor's apartment very eager to be with him. But, despite our attempts at intercourse, Viktor was too well endowed for us to proceed. We were clearly clueless about lube and I was likely not fully aroused. I obviously still had much to learn. Yet, it remained a poignant memory between the two of us.

Now, on this current trip to Florida, Viktor and I were reunited in what felt to be a magical moment, suspended in time. His car arrived in the driveway; he parked, exited the car and saw me standing in wait on the porch. I saw him move towards me. He was pulled to me as if by some invisible thread pulling us together, drawing him closer.

And then I was in his arms, warm encircling arms holding me to him as if never to let go. I felt my heart reaching out and connecting to his. Time stood still. I felt something even greater pulling me to him. A sense of knowing washed over me; I had the sensation that I was coming home after a long journey.

We spent an amazing day together, enjoying each other's company. Later, as the end of the day drew towards its end, I could not bear the thought of saying goodbye. It would be too painful. Thankfully, Viktor suggested that we continue our visit into the night.

After a long drive and time spent on various activities, we were finally alone. Viktor swept me up in his arms and carried me off to his bedroom. He placed me gently on the bed and joined the space next to me. It was then that we decided that this was no longer a fantasy; our love was real and could no longer remain a dream. We had spent a lot of time talking with one another about what could be; it was now time to stop talking and start doing. Nothing else had ever felt so right or made as much sense. We were no longer willing to be apart and we no longer wished to live separate lives. Viktor wanted me in his life as much as I wanted him in mine.

Ready to make the necessary commitments to give our hearts fully to each other, we were confident that our love would bond us forever. In this, we vowed to give our relationship the chance it deserved and were willing to give it all the patience and energy that was required. We stayed up all night talking and sharing and making plans.

Finally, in the last hours of the night, Viktor took me in his arms and together we physically consummated our promise. It was the most beautiful moment when we finally became one. We had shared so much over the past eight years and now we had shared this most precious and intimate experience, which, at the time, felt utterly transcendent. In our hearts, we knew that we had found our partner for life in each other, forsaking all others.

At the end of that vacation, I returned home and told my parents and friends that I was "pre-engaged." I don't know where I got that silly term from, but it was clear that Viktor and I wanted to create a life together. By June, I had given up my apartment in Manhattan, leased a car and moved to Florida to be with Viktor, with the expectation that we would *actually* get engaged and then married. I was excited to be with this man that I loved so much. I had wanted to be with him for so long and we were finally going to be together...for the rest of our lives.

But, upon moving in together, I found myself lacking in desire. What had happened to the sexually empowered woman who had boldly pursued men? Where had my interest in self-pleasure disappeared to? Why was I so shut down? I had just upended my life in New York and moved to someplace in which I knew almost no one, started a job search, then began a new job, all while Viktor worked long, late hours as General Manager of a restaurant. Maybe it was depression; maybe it was the birth control pills.

But I also felt so at odds with being a soon-to-be wife and being a sexual person. Growing up watching too many episodes of *Donna Reed* on "Nick at Nite," I didn't know how to reconcile what it meant to be a spouse and a sexually empowered woman. I had no role model. This identity crisis and the utter loss of libido left me feeling damaged and led me to the therapist's office.

As weeks turned to months, we were having sex only sporadically. I still felt almost no sexual desire for my fiancé or even less interest in self-pleasure. I was convinced that I was "broken" and turned to therapy to "fix" me. I spent a lot of time talking, but with little obvious results. I went on antidepressants[2] and stopped taking the pill, but my libido didn't return. I was at a loss as to how to reignite my sexual passion. Talking about sex with my therapist felt productive in one sense, but there was no real progress to speak of. And talking about sex was uncomfortable; I felt icky. Sex felt icky, shameful. I didn't feel confident and excited about sex; I felt gross.

Viktor and I essentially had a sexless marriage, or at least an under-sexed marriage. I felt guilty about denying him sex and offered for him to find someone else to have sex with. He lovingly declined and we simply went on with our limited sex life.

Two years into our marriage, not much had changed. I desperately wanted to be healed; to be normal. Viktor and I were creating a new sense of intimacy. We communicated more effectively, and I felt much closer to him. I knew that we had progressed, strengthening our relationship, so these improvements were important. Yet, I was unable to let myself go to experience things; to feel things and not just observe things. It was difficult and again and again I pulled back, eventually closing down and shutting off.

We would occasionally plan sex weekends, which somehow worked to permit me to relax, get out of my head and engage in long, overdue sexual activity with Viktor. On one such weekend, I made a note in my journal that we had had what I jokingly referred to as "hat trick sex;" we had had sex three times in one night. This was very novel for us at the time.

But I still didn't own my sexuality; it owned me. One date night, rather than wear typical pantyhose, I chose to wear stockings and a garter belt. But, instead of feeling confident and sexy, I felt shameful and slutty. I found myself sitting at the restaurant's bar tugging at my skirt to cover up and hide the garter belt from anyone's view.

---

[2] Wellbutrin, which thankfully doesn't interfere with libido the way so many other antidepressants do.

On other occasions, I would have a bout of sexual desire such as when we attended a friend's wedding at the botanical garden and hid in some bushes engaging in sexual behavior. But, I awakened the next morning with a double hangover — that of the alcohol and that of the deep discomfort of having been an active participant in sex. Who was that woman that wanted sex? That wasn't me, I thought.

Desperately seeking desire

I was resigned to our life. I loved my husband, and I knew he loved me. We were affectionate, just not overly sexual. I tried to assuage the guilt and simply ignore it all. I continued to go to therapy, but I still didn't feel what I wanted to feel. I knew that I — that we — deserved so much more. But I felt powerless to make a change. Or, rather, I felt powerless in that I didn't know what to do. Despite years of therapy, nothing had really changed.

Then, ten years into our marriage, I found something new to try. I started taking classes at S Factor, a sensual dance movement that pushes women to connect with their erotic nature. I had heard about S Factor a few years before, having seen Sheila Kelley (S Factor's creator) on *Oprah*.

Inspired by the way she felt after starring in and co-producing the movie *Dancing at the Blue Iguana*, Sheila started teaching classes in her Los Angeles home before eventually opening a studio downtown. Other studio locations followed, with a New York location added in 2006 after Gerri Kyhill took a class in California and knew that New York City had to have this incredible experience.

I was initially drawn to S Factor as a way to jumpstart my libido. I had been considering taking belly dancing lessons in lieu of joining a gym, when I learned about the opening of the New York S Factor studio. This seemed like a good way to pursue both aims, so I instantly signed up for an Introductory class.

I immediately fell in love with this interpretation of pole dancing from my very first Intro. But, as much as I loved this "jungle-gym for adults," S Factor was (and is) so much more than pole tricks; it combined elements of yoga, Pilates and sensual movement, along with pole, and, most importantly, encompassed an emotional journey that put a woman in touch with her erotic self.

Strikingly dissimilar to other pole or dance studios, S Factor students danced in rooms without mirrors and to the equivalent of candlelight. It was not about what you looked like, but rather, what you felt like as you moved your body in all of its glorious feminine curves. Through S Factor's unique blend of movement, women were not only invited, but encouraged, to own their sexuality and sensuality and to discover what Sheila calls their EC — their Erotic Creature. There are ten EC icons, based on ten different core emotions that can be expressed, with the belief that every woman possesses all ten icons, but that two or three are the most dominant within her.

Since that first class, I was hooked, learning to really allow my body to express herself as a woman — moving in feminine and sexy ways. Slowing down and relishing my curves; enjoying my body for myself. Expressing rage, expressing joy, embracing lust and eradicating shame. It didn't happen overnight, and, in fact, I recall the discomfort I felt at being asked to bring our hands to our bodies, caressing our curves during the warmup. I was afraid that my fellow classmates would think badly of me in seeing me touch myself in this way. Would they think I was perverted? Yet, deep down, I knew this was important for my sensual growth, so I pushed on.

By July 2008, with two years of S Factor under my belt, I wondered if I was making sufficient (sexual) progress to justify S Factor? I was still extremely uncomfortable with sex and my lack of sexual desire remained. I found myself forcing myself to have sex with Viktor as an attempt to normalize things. But I kept going. The following year, my desire list included: quality sex and increased quantity of sex. Sex (or the lack thereof) continued to be a "problem" for me, but one I was desperate to overcome.

Yet, while my S Factor journey wasn't enough to fully awaken my sexual desire, it was responsible for so much of my progress. Over the past fifteen years of classes, I had made extraordinary discoveries about myself, as I relearned how to move, how to just be and to unabashedly be sexual without fear, guilt or apology. After so many years of self-blame and shame, I finally owned my sexuality and my sensual self.

I felt really pleased about how far I had come, but I still wanted so much more. The "more" next came in the guise of pursuing classes in women's empowerment from a place of pleasure. In 2012, I began studying with Regena Thomashauer at her School of the Womanly Arts, further pushing my boundaries. I had read about Regena, who goes by the moniker, Mama Gena, in a magazine article many years earlier, but I hadn't been taught to invest in personal development programs and the idea of shelling out a lot of money in this direction was very uncomfortable. I finally bit the bullet and signed up for her Virtual Pleasure Boot Camp. It was a good first step, opening me up to the idea of living life from a place of pleasure. This was such a foreign concept for me; like so many women, I was so used to living from a place of pain and fear.

I knew I wanted even more and enrolled in Mama Gena's Mastery course in Spring 2014. The first weekend was transformative. My head was spinning in the days that followed. I knew that this was the next piece of the puzzle and through my work with the School of Womanly Arts and my immersion in the Sister Goddess community, I started to plant seeds, more fully overcoming body shame and stepping more completely into my sexual power.

As I mused about my experiences in the very first Mastery weekend, I wasn't quite sure what I felt. Wow! Whoa! What? Wait a minute, what just happened? A lot. Mind blown, heart open, tuned in, turned on, even a bit turned off. Day one focused on honoring our pussies after a lifetime of shame, embarrassment, fear, disgust and other negative thoughts and attitudes. Despite the fear, I was determined to push through because I knew this was one of the most important areas for me: owning my sexuality and sensuality; taking hold of and standing in my feminine power; banishing fear and shame.

On the Tuesday after the first weekend, I took a mirror and examined my own pussy up close. I saw a Calla Lily. I tried to look past the asymmetry of my labia knowing that it wasn't relevant or important; my pussy was beautiful no matter what. That night I told Viktor that my pussy looked like a Calla Lily while we were having sex. I could feel change bubbling up to the surface.

In the following days, Viktor and I had the most wonderful conversations about what I had been experiencing and we continued to keep that thread of intimacy alive all week. It was evident that the passion missing in our marriage could be revived with love, caring and time. This sparked the first in many conversations that were to follow about our marriage, intimacy and sex life. We continued to talk and revisit this conversation from time to time.

The second weekend of Mastery, students were invited to go to lunch with whomever we wanted. My new-found friend, Kimberly, immediately asked if I wanted to join her and her friend, Ray. I quickly said yes and was so glad I did. Lunch was amazing because we had a very honest discussion about threesomes as well as other sexual issues and desires. This was something I had always wanted to talk about but never had the right audience. I felt exhilarated.

I truly don't remember how Viktor and I first discussed it, but I know that the idea of a threesome came up early in our marriage. At that time, I was deathly afraid of what a single non-monogamous encounter might do to our marriage and wasn't willing to take a chance on one night of sex. Given that frame of mind, I am confident that I made the right decision to abstain from following through.

Now, years, possibly decades, later, as this idea of threesomes, open marriage, etc. came up in the context of this luncheon discussion, I was so thrilled to be at that lunch, having that conversation. Before that, I had never felt comfortable to share these fantasies and desires with anyone other than my husband. I had been so afraid that friends would think that my marriage was in trouble, be concerned that I was hitting on them or be upset that I wasn't.

In many ways, the Mama Gena experience brought about seismic shifts. I had a renewed interest in self-pleasure and in sex in general. Things between Viktor and me became so much better, but despite the progress, I was still not at the place I wanted to be.

A while later, I befriended a woman in my women's community who was frank about her open marriage and on another occasion met a woman who had a husband with a lover and her own lover. It was enlightening and freeing and gave me the impetus to revisit the conversation with Viktor.

In the beginning, I was hesitant to bring up these topics, but I felt compelled to give voice to these desires. Yes, that first conversation was scary, but then, once it was over, I noticed something remarkably interesting: our talk about bringing in other partners was pulling us closer together rather than pushing us apart, as we bared our souls and got intimate in the most vulnerable and honest of ways.

I was also terrified that such a move on either of our parts would potentially damage the beautiful foundation we had built over our decades of marriage. We continued to verbally explore these ideas; sharing what elements were tantalizing, which weren't and what we ultimately wanted from such an exploration. Each time we talked, our foundation grew more solid and I knew that, if and when we were ready to move forward, it would be strong enough to hold us in this next chapter of our journey.

We continued to revisit these conversations in the months and years that followed. They continued to spark intimacy, desire and love with my husband. But, despite the positive nature of these discussions, neither of us was ready to do anything other than talk until several years had passed.

Over the course of our marriage, we had spent countless hours talking about our sex life (or lack thereof) and experienced numerous failed attempts to infuse more sex into our lives. But we also discovered many wins along the way as we studied with somatic sexologist Miss Jaiya, participated in a Tantra class with Barbara Carrellas and explored the D/s world with Om Rupani. But the results of these explorations were short-lived. I wanted to truly step into my sexual self and maintain ongoing sexual desire.

So, over the next four years, Viktor and I had incredible discussions about threesomes and open marriages. But, with each subsequent discussion, we became clearer on what we wanted and felt comfortable with, and most importantly, recognized that we were not going to damage our marriage. We were confident that our marriage was strong enough to sustain whatever this experiment might do. We agreed to keep the dialog constantly open between us, checking in to see what we did or didn't want at each stage of the journey and made the commitment to stop at any time if we decided that it was no longer working.

Throughout this journey, Viktor had been my steadfast supporter, lover and confidante. I had never once doubted that we were meant to be together or wavered in my love for him. By 2017, I felt the hunger so deeply. My top desires were to truly devote myself to my sex life and marriage; to fully release body shame and sex shame; and to fully embrace all of me. I wanted more physical connection with my husband, including sensual connection and desire.

And, yet I still felt stuck. During class one day, my S Factor instructor asked me point blank: "What is your desire? How do you want to be fucked?" I was struck by a ball of sadness at not knowing the answer and anger at myself for having got to this place. I wanted to know; I *had* to know. If I didn't know, how could I possibly expect Viktor to know?

I was at the end of my rope not knowing what else to do anymore — desperately wanting something that seemed to come so easily and natural to everyone else to the point that they were risking marriages, life, etc. and I couldn't find the desire despite loving my husband so much. I knew something more had to happen.

It was time...

Part Two

The Summer of Sexiness: Down the Rabbit Hole

In 2018, still dissatisfied with my level of sexual desire, Viktor and I agreed to embark on a new chapter as we explored the ins and outs of an open relationship. In early May of that year, I went to an erotic party with my friend Tova, hosted by our mutual friend Serafina. Both of us were nervous and excited to attend, not knowing what to expect or what we wanted out of the evening. I just knew that I wanted to be open to new experiences and to really participate, not just watch from the sidelines. In keeping with that intention, I used the event's pink pleasure theme as an excuse to purchase a new set of sexy lingerie. I also knew that I didn't want to have sex with a stranger. But did I want to connect with anyone? And, if so, to what extent did I want to engage?

Soon after we arrived, Tova and I met Hank who gave each guest a tour of the space and introduced folks to one another. Shortly thereafter, the party got underway. First, Serafina welcomed everyone to the event with a beautiful ritual and then, she and her partner demonstrated the concept of enthusiastic consent — a critical element to the party. At this point, the party was set in motion.

Where did I wish to start? The people engaging in sex off to the side seemed to be having fun, but I had no desire to join them. And I wasn't sure that I desired to be flogged. As I was standing and talking with Tova, Hank came over and asked if he could touch my arm. I said yes. It felt nice. He then asked if he could massage my neck. I said yes again and that also felt nice; very nice, in fact. Next, Hank asked if he could kiss me. I froze for a second. I hadn't kissed anyone other than my husband in more than 20 years. In that moment, it was a clear no, which I communicated to him while thanking him for his interest.

Hank continued to gently touch and massage me with my consent. We then walked over to the corner of the room where a massage table was set up, making it easier for me to relax into the massage. Then, at my invitation, Hank climbed onto the table with me. Feeling bolder and more at ease with him, I gave him permission to touch me in a more sexually explicit way as well as permission to kiss me.

It was very erotic and alluring, as I felt his attention on me and his desire for me. It was a heady aphrodisiac. While we were kissing, he said, "I can't wait to taste you," which sent shivers of electricity through me and continued to do so every time I thought about it in the week that followed. I definitely wasn't ready for oral sex with someone new, but the statement was extremely arousing!

After our make-out session, Hank asked for my phone number, which I gave him, and he asked if he could take me to dinner to which I replied maybe. He texted me right away so I would have his number, but I waited until the next evening to reply. I wanted to see if I was still interested before I encouraged further interactions.

The day after the party I shared the whole story with Viktor, who was very turned on by what he heard. As I spoke, I felt that I was still buzzing with the energy from the night before; I felt feverish and untethered. Once I concluded my tale, Viktor began to kiss me intensely, touching my breasts and further igniting my turn-on until he pleasured me to orgasm. It was evident that this first foray into the unknown world of an open marriage was a positive one for us and was having its desired result, helping me explore my turn-on and enhancing our sexual intimacy.

After our initial meeting at the party, Hank and I texted back and forth during the week, eventually setting up dinner plans. As I counted down the days to our date, I was excited and filled with wonder. All week I hummed with energetic arousal like never before. I still felt ungrounded, yet alive, aflame! It was amazing and exhausting all at once.

Plus, there was the anticipation of a first date after 20-plus years. What should I wear? What would I say? And, more importantly, what did I want? As I got dressed, I texted with Tova who asked me what my desires for the date might be. I told her that I wanted to have an open and honest conversation with Hank, get to know him better and feel out what might be possible for our non-conventional relationship. I desired to feel his desire; to feel his gaze and attention; and for him to sensually kiss me on the back of my neck. Then, I headed out the door and was on my way.

I met Hank at a Japanese restaurant as planned, dressed in an LBD (little black dress), fishnet stockings and 5-inch heels, feeling beautiful and sexy. Our initial interactions were awkward at first, as we were both nervous and unsure what to expect, but I soon felt comfortable in his presence and was delighted to note that my desire for him was still there. I enjoyed his compliments and his gaze as we talked over dinner.

As we finished our meal, Hank expressed his interest in continuing to spend time with me that evening, and explicitly mentioned that he wanted to kiss the back of my neck. I had just explained desire lists with him 30 minutes earlier and practically blew his mind when I showed him my text to Tova!

With our mutually agreed upon agenda (having him kiss my neck), we looked for a dark bar in which to connect more intimately. We found a dive bar, which wasn't quite as dark as we had hoped, but decided that it was fine for our purposes. We sat at the bar, engaging in inappropriate behavior — kissing and caressing each other in full view of other patrons (don't judge!) — before calling it a night. While such public displays of affection weren't usually my style, it was really thrilling to be kissing him so intently and it was quite a turn-on.

As we said goodbye, we shared our mutual desire for future encounters and talked about possible plans for the upcoming holiday weekend. I was intrigued by where it might lead, especially as Hank expressed some willingness to engage in a threesome with Viktor and me.

Arriving home after the date, Viktor was still up, so I briefed him on my date. He was genuinely happy for me and we both felt the turn-on of the evening, choosing to channel it into a sexual liaison. So far, Hank was having an incredibly positive influence on our marriage!

After that first date with Hank, our texting morphed into sexting, which was a new experience for me — my previous dating experiences were in the olden (aka pre-cellphone) days. Hearing my phone chime with the arrival of his sexts became almost Pavlovian as I became aroused by his missives expressing his desire to kiss me all over, taste my wetness and share an erotic dream he had had.

But it was clear that we both wanted to move things from the virtual to the actual, so Hank and I arranged to meet up on the Friday of Memorial Day weekend for a picnic. He suggested that we could pick up sandwiches and some wine when I got to his neighborhood, but I texted back that I had a much different picnic in mind. Rather, I was imagining a sensual picnic with strawberries, blueberries, whipped cream, and chocolate. He immediately acquiesced to the new plan and even asked me which kind of whipped cream he should buy.

On the day of our date, Hank met me at his subway stop and then we headed to Brooklyn Bridge Park together and found the perfect picnic spot. Once we were settled on our blanket, we slowly fed each other fresh berries topped with whipped cream and luscious chocolates, pausing between bites to enjoy sips of the dessert wine I had brought. And, when not eating, we were deliciously kissing. About two hours later we packed up our picnic and walked to Hank's apartment.

Once in his apartment, we were finally free to be more explicit with our kisses, touches and body exploration and we were soon both naked. Having stated that he couldn't wait to taste me when we first met, it was no surprise when Hank shifted his attention from my lips and breasts to my clitoris. But, despite wanting the experience, it didn't feel quite right as I wasn't fully relaxed and felt pressure to climax quickly, so I asked him to stop.

Hank was very reassuring that there was no pressure or rush to do anything I didn't want to do and instead returned to kissing me elsewhere. We spent several hours engaged in sensual play, occasionally pausing to talk and share. Still a bit awkward and shy with a new partner, I wasn't ready to give him head, even though I had researched safer sex and blowjobs in advance of our date, but did give him a handjob, truly feeling into what I wanted (and what I didn't want). It was wonderful and freeing.

We eventually decided we were hungry (fruit, whipped cream and chocolate are yummy, but not entirely filling) and went to dinner at Hank's favorite local spot with a fabulous view of the sunset and the Manhattan skyline. Earlier he had asked me about what else was on my desire list and I admitted that I had something on the list that was too far-fetched to share at this juncture, but after several playful requests from him and a few cocktails later, I finally shared it: to pole dance for him and my husband on my birthday and then have them whisk me away to a fancy hotel room and have their way with me. Plus, lots of sparkling wine and cake. He didn't flinch!

After dinner, we returned to his apartment, spent some more time kissing and then he called an Uber for me, saw me into the car and had me text him when I got home. It was the perfect ending to a lovely day.

During our Friday date, I had mentioned that I was visiting a friend on Monday (Memorial Day) who lived near him. He said that if she and I planned to meet in the neighborhood, I should let him know, since he would love to see me again. After I confirmed plans with my friend, I reached out to Hank to see if he was still up for seeing me on Monday and he said yes. We arranged that I would come by with smoked salmon and have brunch together in his home.

He again met me at the subway and walked me to his apartment. Once there, I offered to dance for him, guiding him to sit in his armchair for a good view. I then turned on some music and moved slowly and sensually, peeling off my leggings and dress and giving him a brief lap dance. As the song ended, Hank took my hand and led me to his bed, resuming our make-out session from Friday. While we were in bed, I was much more relaxed this time and was truly able to surrender to his touch and tongue in orgasm. A few hours later, I met up with my friend Lanie.

After spending time with her, I returned home to Viktor who had been away all weekend and filled him in on my adventures with Hank. He was so turned on and took me to bed where we created our own adventure.

After our marathon Memorial Day Weekend date, I didn't hear from Hank much and the week that followed was quiet and uneventful in that regard. Then I departed for a work trip to Italy, during which time texts from Hank were limited at best and I began to question his interest in what we were doing. I was unwilling to chase him and instead waited to see what would happen. We finally made plans for the weekend of Serafina's next erotic party, but his attention was still a bit lackluster and our actual plans were only half formed, so I was admittedly anxious as the date drew near.

Since Viktor was out of town on business, I had invited Hank to come to my apartment and welcomed him to stay the night. He had initially invited me to stay over at his place after the party, but it wasn't feasible due to dog obligations (and Viktor's absence) and, moreover, I wanted an actual date, not just a hook-up/sleeping session after the party. Always a planner by nature, I had several options in my head and was prepared with a range of ideas including a picnic (more extensive than last time), a visit to my local wine bar or simply staying in.

Upon his arrival, Hank was conscientious of my neighbors and did not kiss me in the lobby, but quickly rectified this upon entering my home, wherein our dog immediately started to bark at him. She eventually settled down, but it was very funny, and I later related to Viktor that she had his back. I gave Hank a tour of the apartment, except for the master bedroom, the door to which was closed, protecting the sanctity of that space.

Collectively, Hank and I had decided that it was too cold for a picnic and instead sat on the couch kissing and then soon moved to the guest room, promptly embarking on an intense make-out session, progressing from kisses to caresses and then removing our clothes. He was very much in awe of my Agent Provocateur lingerie. I felt a moment of power as he exclaimed, "Fuck" as I unzipped my skirt and slowly pulled my shirt over my head and he saw me in just the bra and panties.

As we began to engage in sensual play, I reminded him that we had talked about playing with toys together, so after a brief sojourn for some wine (aka liquid courage), we returned to the bedroom to explore. I pleasantly relaxed into his presence as I used the vibrator on myself, focusing on my clit and eventually bringing myself to orgasm. Then, after rummaging through my pleasure basket, Hank expressed interest in being gently handcuffed and blindfolded, as he had never engaged in this type of play before. Once the restraints were in place, I selected a feather and teased him with it, then kissed his neck, chest, stomach and thighs before touching his cock.

After our play session, we stopped to enjoy a late dinner, along with more of the wine. Then, we decided it was time to go to bed, lying naked and entangled in each other's arms, which I found to be more alluring in theory than in practice. But, despite the lack of a restful night's sleep, I did enjoy the freedom of being so vulnerable and intimate with him.

Upon waking, we walked the dog, and I gave Hank a tour of the nearby park, since he had expressed interest and had also enjoyed sharing his neighborhood with me. For breakfast, I made blueberry pancakes and Hank helped to fry the bacon. We returned to bed for more cuddling and then Hank went down on me properly this time. I was able to relax and enjoy his attention, feeling the pleasurable sensations throughout my body.

Still not ready to engage in a blowjob or intercourse, I give him a handjob and eventually he used the friction of my body to cum. We showered together, sudsing each other with soap and then, once dry and dressed, watched the documentary, *My Erotic Body*, because it features S Factor and I wanted to share that part of myself with him. By then, it was 1:00 p.m. and Hank headed home, knowing that we would see each other that night at the erotic party.

Return to the scene of the sublime

Since I had really enjoyed my first erotic party, I was eager to attend this same event, now a month later. And, while I had always known that Hank would also be at the party, my decision to attend was based solely on my own desires. So, while I did look forward to spending time with him, I also hoped to meet other people and press new edges.

Hank had talked about us playing together with some other (unknown) woman with me sitting on his face, while instructing her to give him a blowjob, but how such a scene would come to fruition was nebulous and I expressed equal parts potential interest and trepidation.

I took my time getting ready for the party, indulging in a bubble bath, carefully choosing my lingerie and outfit, and getting into the theme: A Midsummer's Night Dream. Inspired by another friend who had noted that she would be sporting fairy wings, I chose to don a floral crown, putting it on at home and wearing it on the journey instead of waiting to get to the party. I felt sexy, beautiful and alive as I headed to Brooklyn.

After transferring from one subway line to another, I noticed that the man sitting next to me on the train looked familiar and I thought he was someone I had met at the previous party. But, how to know for sure? Talking to strangers on the subway was already a bit dicey, but to ask if someone had been at an erotic party would really be bold (and potentially dangerous). We both disembarked the train at the same stop and after acknowledging that we were both looking for the same address, the recognition was mutually confirmed. His name was Tim.

Tim and I arrived at the venue and ventured into what would be a magical night. I headed downstairs and was greeted by Hank, who was once again helping to co-host the event and was thus busy for the early part of the evening.

Hanging out at the bar, I met Kevin, who admired my crown and began to flirt with me a bit. I enjoyed the banter and attention but did feel a little torn as I wanted to reconnect with Hank after our previous night's date, but also wanted to be open to new experiences and to see what else might happen. I could feel how being noticed (via the crown) made me feel desired and seen.

After Kevin drifted off, I spent time talking with friends and then chatted with a guy who referred to himself as BK Dom. Somehow, we ended up talking about bike racing, a sport in which Viktor is highly active and I never got to find out about his other "passions," still left wondering if BK Dom meant that he was a Dominant (as in Dominant/submissive) or simply a guy from Brooklyn named Dominic.

Also, as he wandered away in search of others, I thought about the etiquette of mentioning a husband, especially since I never explained that we had an open marriage. I had intentionally not worn my wedding ring (not to deliberately mislead anyone, but to ensure that I was approachable and didn't appear to be off-limits, but it was an awkward and confusing dance that I realized I would have to learn to negotiate on this new journey.

Only slightly disappointed, I, too, veered away from the bar, finding Hank and walking through the downstairs area watching people in various acts of sexual play. It was titillating to watch, but I still didn't feel any compulsion to participate. Being honest with myself, I realized that, at least at this stage, I would be unable to relax enough to enjoy myself in the presence of so many people.

Hank and I headed back outside, settling onto the couch near the fire pit, where we watched people getting tied up by a Shibari (Japanese rope bondage) master. Ahead of time, I had decided that I wanted to participate in this activity since I hadn't done so last time, but, once at the party, I didn't necessarily want to wait on what seemed to be a lengthy line. Instead, I sat back and savored the show as rope was intricately wound around the human form.

A short while later, Hank introduced me to his friends Jake and Mia, who he knew from when he used to throw swingers' parties. They joined us on the couch, and we talked about the rope scene among other things. Then Jake asked if I had ever been tied up. "No." Had I ever been chained? Again, I responded, "No." Would I like to be? "Wait, what? You mean now?" He did mean now and then suddenly I was up on the balcony with Jake and Mia.

A leather collar was fastened around my neck, joined by restraints on my wrists, which were then linked by chains to the collar. They put a blindfold over my eyes and asked for permission to pull my bodysuit down, exposing my breasts. I consented and then Jake asked if my breasts were overly sensitive. I wasn't sure how to answer but admitted that I had never used nipple clamps. We agreed that I was willing to try a soft clamp and Jake attached it to my left breast. It pinched, but it was more of a discomfort than actual pain. Then, a flood of sensations followed...from all sides. I felt breath, I felt kisses, I felt my nipples being fondled. I couldn't see or tell who was touching me anymore and I didn't care. It felt wonderful and exciting and overwhelming. Then, I began to feel lightheaded and let Jake know that I regretfully needed to stop (but I figured that stopping was way sexier than passing out!).

After removing the cuffs, collar, clamp and blindfold, Mia brought me some water and I took some time to rest, reconnecting with Hank for a bit. A while later I was introduced to a random guy by an acquaintance. There was an instant connection as he slathered on the compliments. I felt his penetrating gaze and liked it. I felt super sexy and in control. As we sat on the couch, he asked me what my deal was, and I shared where I was at. He questioned me about Hank, but I assured him that there was no need to worry about Hank; it was up to me to decide whom I wanted to be with at any given time.

In between kisses, the random guy and I continued to talk, and he seemed more and more intrigued as I disclosed different details of myself. I felt energized by his adoration of these things that made me precisely and uniquely me. I liked the idea that who I am was so alluring and I tried to hold onto this sensation and knowledge as he told me I was perfect. He also revealed that he was very into oral sex, which I got him to clarify meant that he loved to give it.

He further expressed that he had the patience to give it for hours. I was quite intrigued and frankly a bit tempted, but as I had acknowledged to myself earlier, I wouldn't feel comfortable to participate in such an overt sexual experience in a party environment. I wondered if we could plan on something for another night but discovered that he was visiting from out of town for the weekend only, so there was no way to explore our connection further and chose to put an end to our encounter.

Once up and off the couch, I stumbled across Hank who said that he was getting ready to head home. I felt a little guilty for ignoring him a bit but tried to push those thoughts aside as we certainly didn't have any exclusive access to each other, not to mention the whole swingers' lifestyle was essentially about sharing (yes, there was much more to it than that, but I figured he had experience in this regard).

As I was speaking with Hank, Jake came up to me, letting me know that he and Mia were also about to leave and offered me a ride home. I decided that I was "full" from the party and accepted his invitation. I went to say goodbye to the random man, explaining that I had a ride home. He asked me to stay and noted that he would pay for a ride home later, but I kindly declined, kissed him one last time and wished him well.

I followed Jake and Mia back downstairs toward the exit, where I saw Kevin and let him know I was leaving. He expressed interest in seeing me again and also offered me a ride home if I wanted to stay longer, but I gave him my business card instead and encouraged him to contact me.

Once outside, Jake and Mia asked if I was in a hurry to get home (I wasn't) and asked me if I would join them for dinner. I would. They took me to a restaurant in Chinatown, where we talked about my experience with them and my interest in repeating it in the future as well as having a more general discussion of the swingers' lifestyle. Then, they drove me home and kissed me goodbye, before I headed into my apartment and off to bed.

I awoke early the next morning, a bit dazed, thinking about the party's opening ritual during which the question had been posed: "Was it really a dream or was it reality?" A slew of texts from Hank, Jake and Kevin in the hours that followed all provided evidence to the latter...as did my Chinese cookie fortune that read, "Stay in touch, above all, with how you feel."

Over the next two weeks, I texted back and forth with Jake and Mia. They had initially invited me to join them at a swingers' party, but I had another commitment on that date, and we agreed that it would be better to connect as a threesome, rather than at a party, given my newness to the lifestyle.

We finally confirmed a date for an upcoming Friday. That Friday morning, they advised me that they would get a hotel room in New Jersey (they lived in New Jersey) and then would text me the room number. I had always fantasized about participating in a threesome and really looked forward to sharing the experience with them. I spent the afternoon leisurely getting ready — bubble bath, primping, beautifying — and tried not to get too nervous.

I Googled "What to bring to a threesome," but other than condoms, nothing else was mentioned. I eventually chose to bring condoms, lube, a robe, a bottle of Bordeaux, corkscrew and three plastic cups, none of which turned out to be needed (they had their own lube and didn't really drink wine). Half joking, half serious, I next Googled, "What to wear to a threesome," but got no hits. Accordingly, I selected a beautiful lingerie set; a clingy, black dress, which would be easy to take off (no zippers, buttons, etc.); and a pair of black dress sandals (but nothing too high since I knew I had to walk half a mile from the bus to the hotel).

Once I was at the hotel, I took the elevator upstairs, arrived at their door, knocked and was immediately ushered into the candle-lit room by Jake and Mia. They poured me a vodka and coke, which I gratefully accepted. They then directed me to remove my dress and bra so that Jake could give me a massage to help me relax. Jake rubbed oil onto my back and began to gently massage my muscles, but eventually turned me over, at which point Mia joined in, slowly massaging my breasts and ultimately kissing them.

From there, things got more heated and Mia asked if they could tie me up again (as they had at the party). I consented and out came the collar, wrist cuffs and chain. While they adorned my body, blindfolded me and began to stimulate me, they used my phone to take photos of the experience to share with Viktor. It was an incredible experience, being the sole focus of their dual attention, with the diverse stimulation and sensual/sexual touch and play. Mia used a vibrator on me, bringing to climax.

Then, I returned the favor, as she and Jake were fucking, I applied the vibrator on her clit, adding a clitoral orgasm to her experience. Later in the evening, I spent one-on-one time playing with Mia (being with a woman was another long-held fantasy) and then, still later, with Jake. Around 1:30 a.m., they invited me to spend the night. I agreed, texted Viktor not to expect me until morning and climbed into bed, with Jake between Mia and me.

The next morning, I woke to Jake and Mia having sex and then there was more kissing, fondling and groping among the three of us, but for the most part, we packed up and they drove me home. Once home, I shared my experience with Viktor, handed him the phone so he could see the photos and then he took me to bed, so I could be properly fucked (despite the intensity and intimacy of our encounter, I had chosen not to have intercourse with Jake).

A few weeks later, I had my first date with Kevin whom I had also met at the second erotic party. Our evening was relatively tame, but still nice. We met at a casual restaurant overlooking the Hudson River, with views of the sunset.

Over drinks and a light dinner, we had a lovely time getting to know one another and feeling each other out for what we were looking for. It seemed like he wanted to take things slowly, build a connection and was just generally a sweet guy. I wondered if perhaps he might be too nice/too vanilla but was open to see what would happen with time. And I really liked his flirty texts; he had sent me a photo of his pool and noted that bathing suits were not permitted at night.

During dinner, he complimented me and used the specific word — stunning — that I had written on my desire list for the date. After dinner, we walked along the river in the park, stopping to kiss for a long time. They were very tantalizing kisses and I enjoyed being held by him. Then he drove me home (which had been another written desire).

After that first date, Kevin and I made plans to meet up a few weeks later. I didn't hear from him much after that and my interest in him waned a bit as a result. But, the week of the scheduled date, I texted him to see if we were still on and he said yes. Since he lived on Long Island, we arranged for me to take the train out east on a Friday evening, but left the specific plans a bit vague.

While I was on the train, Kevin texted that he had made a restaurant reservation and asked if that was okay with me. I replied that it was, secretly pleased that he was stepping up and making the effort since I had felt a little less wanted due to the limited contact and his need to truncate our initial plans due to commitments with his kids. I certainly understood and respected that his kids came first, but I wanted (and needed) to feel special and desired in these relationships.

Upon arrival, Kevin met me at the train station and then drove us into town for dinner. We dined at an Argentine restaurant, catching up a bit and getting to know one another better. Afterward, we headed to a wine bar in the neighboring town, enjoying a glass of wine and flirting with each other. We chose to stop at one glass and then returned to his home. Once inside, he gave me a tour and then opened a bottle of wine.

We took our glasses to Kevin's bedroom and began to sip our wine, but they were soon forgotten as he unzipped and took off my dress, pushed me back on the bed and began to kiss me, really kiss me. Next, he stopped briefly to admire my lingerie and my body, before he unhooked my bra, removing it and my panties. Adjusting me further up on the bed, he started to kiss my nipples, then my stomach and then proceeded to lick my pussy, just as I had desired. It felt really good, but I wasn't fully relaxed and turned on yet.

Shortly after, he paused and took off his clothes. We resumed kissing and then suddenly he surprised me by attempting to have intercourse. Admittedly, we should have had this conversation earlier, but since our first date, and his comments about sex, had seemed relatively tame, I was under the (mistaken) impression that he had wanted to take things more slowly. Clearly, I was wrong. I politely stopped him and explained that I was not yet ready to have penetrative sex with anyone other than my husband and he complied with my wishes.

Instead, we continued to kiss and touch one another, turning each other on and enjoying the co-mingling of our bodies. Sometime later, I jokingly asked him if he still had his handcuffs (he was a retired police-detective). He did. We agreed that it was too soon for me to fully trust being handcuffed but acknowledged that I had liked it when he had held my wrists down tightly earlier in the evening. He asked if I was willing to be tied up and blindfolded and I immediately consented, so he went to retrieve some neckties to repurpose. He initially tied my wrists together, but then we decided it was better to tie each wrist to the bed.

With my eyes blindfolded and arms secured to the bed, he licked and sucked my breasts and my clitoris, not quite pushing me over, but definitely keeping me near the edge of orgasm for some time. It was delicious and exquisite and felt amazing. I loved the feeling of being subdued, making it easier for me to surrender. I still couldn't fully surrender, likely due to us not knowing each other very well, but it was a wonderful experience, nonetheless.

Eventually, we turned off the lights and went to sleep. I dozed throughout the night, alternating between being held in his arms and rolling over on my side to try to actually sleep. Several hours later, the early morning light filtered in through the windows, rousing us from our slumber. Once awake, we resumed our sexual play, then showered together. He made me coffee and an English muffin before he drove me back to the city and walked me to my door, leaving his touch on my body and his kiss on my lips.

Once inside our apartment, I headed to bed for a brief nap, knowing that Viktor and I had a late night ahead with more sexy encounters.

The full swap

To that end, while I wasn't sure what I did "right" on my date with Jake and Mia, I clearly didn't do anything "wrong" since they were eager to see me again. I knew that Viktor was happy for me to have had the threesome with them, but I also got the sense that he would be a little annoyed (and understandably envious) if I saw them again without him. Plus, I knew that he was tired of being a spectator in this "sport" and was ready to participate!

During our texts to set up our date, Jake wanted to know if this would be a Full or Soft swap. Viktor and I had agreed that if I was comfortable and willing to pursue intercourse with Jake, then he was on board with this plan. We both felt that losing my "virginity" this second time to Jake was a good idea given my previous positive experience with him and Mia. Accordingly, I texted back: Full. I was sure that he would be pleased.

Having decided that what you wear to a foursome is fairly similar to what you wear to a threesome, I wasn't as nervous about selecting my outfit this time. I chose a black sundress that required me to skip a bra since I knew Jake didn't really care about lingerie and a G-string panty with a bow, wrapping myself up as a gift to him and Mia.

Again, Jake and Mia had booked a hotel room for us and we planned to meet for drinks in the hotel bar, so that I could introduce Viktor to them, and we could all spend time unwinding and connecting. We arrived a little early, catching them in the lobby and thus went up to the room together, but not before Jake, and then Mia, kissed me hello.

After entering the room, we set up candles, speakers and sex toys. As Mia showered, Jake began to kiss me again, sliding his hand under the halter of my sundress, appreciating the lack of a bra and easy access to my breasts. Suddenly, he turned to Viktor and asked, "Is it okay that I am kissing your wife?" Not waiting for Viktor's response, I laughed and noted that that ship had sailed.

Once the room and its inhabitants were ready, we headed upstairs to the bar, ordering a round of drinks and light bites, which permitted Viktor to get to know Jake and Mia and vice versa since this was the first time they were all meeting. We quickly lapsed into an easy comfort with one another and it was clear that all was a go.

About an hour later, we returned to the room, excited to indulge in our mutual play. Viktor began to kiss Mia as Jake turned his attention to me and soon untied my halter, unzipped my dress and slid it off. As we settled into our respective partners and the evening at hand, Jake licked and teased my nipples, turning me on, before proceeding to give me oral sex. As I climaxed, I offered up my body to Jake, who then put on a condom and began to fuck me.

While the details of the night are a little hazy, it was essentially a wonderfully long, repeated round of oral sex followed by intercourse, coupled with the use of a vibrator, all resulting in multiple orgasms. This was interspersed with touches from Mia and Viktor, further adding to the various stimuli pleasurably assaulting my senses.

Although I found my clitoral orgasms to be the most satisfying, I was amazed at how intense and pleasurable intercourse with Jake was. He was clearly very talented and knowledgeable as he carefully positioned his cock to touch and reach different spots within my pussy. Whereas I had been so concerned about not being able to climax the night before on my date with Kevin, I had no such problem with Jake and was quite vocal in my pleasure. Plus, I had taken edibles to help me relax and get out of my head and it really seemed to work.

Given all of our activities, it was a late night when Viktor and I finally said goodnight to Jake and Mia, heading to bed around 3:00 a.m. Not surprisingly, I woke the next morning quite tired, but truly feeling blissed out and spent.

Tell me what you want

Only a few months into this journey, I was already starting to have a much better sense of what I desired. My experiences with Kevin and Jake had provided me with a clearer glimpse of what I might want. I reveled in the sweetness of surrender; in the joy of letting go and just being, remaining fully in my body and not in my head; lingering in the depth of desire. I took great delight in being possessed by another; by giving myself over to the masculine energy; opening up with wild abandon; absent of fear, anxiety or any power struggle. I wanted to feel all of this coupled with the height of ecstasy; riding wave after wave of orgasm, culminating in pure bliss and contentment.

Yet, I still felt empty and incomplete. I was convinced that there was more to the story; more to what I needed to truly be possessed; to let go completely and fully, without effort. There was still a lingering sadness as I waited for the answer, but I was buoyed with hope as this journey continued to unfold and teach me so much about myself, my body and my desire.

Clearly, meeting Hank had truly kicked off this whole "Summer of Sexiness." It was as if I had been awakened from a long sexless slumber and now felt more alive, more turned on than ever before. I was so excited to receive his texts and really looked forward to our dates and sexual encounters.

And, early on, he had expressed genuine interest in me, making me feel wanted and desired. He also alluded to possible future plans and treated me very well, meeting me at the subway, making sure I got home safely and otherwise ensuring that I felt cared for and cared about.

But, as time went on, the texts grew further and further apart and were vague and less sexy. He would frequently state that "We will make that happen" about something, but then wouldn't be direct about asking me out or trying to schedule a date to *actually* make it happen. I began to feel like I was chasing him and, at one point, even thought he was ghosting me and was minutes away from sending a text to call him out on his disappearance when he finally reached out to say hello. This wasn't the fun, alluring experience I had envisioned or expected. Yet, I still wanted things to work, so I decided to overlook the lack of communication.

Plus, during our initial conversations, Hank appeared eager to learn more about Tantra and other sexually related topics, having not had any previous experience in those topics. We had talked about me serving as his sensual muse, an idea which he seemed to like. Unfortunately, none of this transpired. And I was always the one to orchestrate our dates, suggesting themes such as the sensual picnic, doing a strip tease for him and playing with sex toys together. The situation was losing some of its luster.

Then, our date to go to the New York Botanical Gardens was changed first due to the extreme heat, but then cancelled due to illness on Hank's part. We finally rescheduled our date a few weeks later, but it wasn't an actual date as much as it was a sexual encounter. He came over, we made out and engaged in oral sex. Afterward, he did note that he was hungry and took me out for drinks and tapas at our local Spanish restaurant. But, in my opinion, it was more a date by accident than by design. I began to question if I still wanted a relationship with him.

A week or so later, he texted to say that he was thinking that a 69 might be fun. I agreed. He replied, "We should make it happen," to which I asked why he so frequently used that expression rather than being direct. He suggested that it meant the same thing as "When are you free?" I advised him that it wasn't but did send him some possible dates and we picked a day to meet.

Almost two full weeks went by without any contact from him and then he texted to say hello and confirm if we were still on for that week as scheduled. When I asked him what the plans were, he simply noted that he was done with work at 1:30 p.m. and asked if he should come uptown to my apartment and also asked if I were going to S Factor that evening. In other words, he wasn't going to suggest any plans other than coming over for the 69 he wanted in between his work schedule and my departure for dance class.

I decided that this felt too much like a "booty call" than a real date and also felt very disconnected from him due to the lack of communication. I told him that I thought we should cancel given that I would be up late the night before and getting up early the day of our plans. But I really knew that it was over and wanted to be honest with him.

So, I texted him the next day and shared that things weren't progressing as I had expected when we first started dating and that I wanted and deserved more. I didn't know that he fully understood what I was saying, but he did acknowledge my text graciously and we parted on good terms. Plus, I realized that there were other things about him that would never change, so he could never truly be what or who I wanted from him.

While I didn't regret my decision to say goodbye to Hank, I had started to think that I was asking for too much — such as we women are often conditioned to think — but then my friend Dan modeled exactly the behavior I was looking for when we met up for dinner and drinks one week. So, it confirmed that what I wanted was definitely doable and reasonable.

In one way, I was sorry to see this relationship end as it was not only so promising from the beginning, but also because it was the initial spark to this journey and for that I would be forever grateful. But I was equally grateful for this experience, which had given me the opportunity to learn so much about myself and about what I did (and didn't) want. It was to be the first of many such experiences on this journey.

Yes, in many ways, this journey was about sex, but I was recognizing that I wanted these relationships to be more holistic experiences. I wanted to be wooed; I wanted to be worshipped; I wanted to be wanted and desired. And, while I was not looking to fall in love with anyone, I still craved a connection as well. So, Hank's chapter came to a close and I eagerly awaited to see what the next one had in store for me.

In search of pleasure

Interestingly, when one's summer included threesomes and swaps, you almost forget that you had a sexy weekend when it was just you and your husband (or at least I temporarily forgot when asked about my weekend on a Monday night). But, in fact, it was truly a pleasure to finally perform a sensual dance for Viktor in my new boots. At S Factor, we were encouraged to experiment with clothing, shoes, music and other aspects to coax out our innate Erotic Creature as well as to see which elements helped or hindered in this regard. For some, it might be slinky lingerie, while for others it could be a sparkly tutu or a length of chain.

When I first started with S Factor, I bought a pair of clear stripper heels (because I decided that the clear would match more things than black or red and you always want to be practical when buying stripper heels). Anyway, I never really loved them and eventually tossed them out and replaced them with other high heels.

But it wasn't until that June that I finally took the plunge and invested in a pair of black, thigh-high, patent leather stiletto boots. From the first time I tried them on, they were magical and transformed the way I walked and moved in my dance. I had shared stories of these class experiences with Viktor, but he hadn't seen them in action until we made a specific date for me to dance for him for our upcoming date night.

The plan was to eat a light dinner, take an edible and then I would begin to dance for him before the pot kicked in. I put together a playlist with five songs and settled Viktor onto the chair in our bedroom with a perfect view of the pole. With such a lengthy list of music, I worried that he might get bored, but afterwards he assured me that he enjoyed every minute of it. When the playlist was over, I removed the boots and Viktor led me to the bed and proceeded to finish the strip tease I had started on the dance floor.

Once I was fully nude, Viktor parted my legs and dove down to taste me, expressing his delight with the intensity of my scent (it had been a hot and humid day on which I had taken an S Factor class and walked quite a bit in addition to my dance for Viktor). I had been a little concerned about whether I was still fresh, but apparently Viktor shared the same preference as Napoleon who supposedly urged Josephine not to bathe before he returned to her. Regardless, I really enjoyed seeing Viktor derive such pleasure from me and felt both empowered and sexy that my scent was so intoxicating to him.

After he had sufficiently turned me on, Viktor kissed me and proceeded to pull some rope out from behind the pillow and tied my hands together, which was an unrehearsed, yet a perfect reply to my last song selection, which was "Tie Me Down" by Gryffin & Elley Duhé. By now the pot was in effect and I was fully relaxed and able to surrender to Viktor. Having watched me have sex with Jake, Viktor took a cue from that experience and experimented with different positions, which resulted in an intense, non-clitoral orgasm. While I was still trying to figure out what I was experiencing during these sessions, I was now really intrigued by the idea of a cervical orgasm as well as a Goddess Spot orgasm and was doing some research on this[3].

---

[3] Sex coach Layla Martin has great YouTube videos on these topics.

As I continued to explore my orgasm and my turn-on and felt into my body, the more connected I felt to Viktor as we shared these sexual experiences together. I felt much freer to be open and honest in the bedroom in a way that I had never felt before. While it wasn't one specific thing that had changed, I did feel that I had given myself permission and that seemed to be a critical piece as I found my way and found my pleasure.

Another pleasure research project centered on attending an event with my friend, Gigi. In July, Gigi and I decided to go to the House of Love: Animal event. Held at House of Yes, a venue in the Bushwick neighborhood of Brooklyn, these House of Love events were quasi-fetish parties and provided guests with an opportunity to dress up and slightly explore the fetish world.

While not a true fetish club (and more R-rated compared to the more explicit erotic parties I had attended earlier that summer), it was a great dance party, with fun activities and an edgier (read sexier) vibe than their usual dance parties. If nothing else there was a frisson in the air that encouraged people to be open to new experiences. For me, these parties provided the perfect backdrop in which to flit from one scene to another all in the name of conducting pleasure research as I experimented with different stimuli.

In keeping with the evening's theme, I dressed in an animal print bodysuit, tulle mini-skirt, fishnet stockings, a pair of 5-inch heels and reprised my floral crown from the Midsummer Night's Party the month before. Arriving a little after 11:00 p.m. on a Saturday night, Gigi and I immediately hit the dimly lit dance floor and shortly thereafter an exotic-looking guy started dancing with me.

I was pleased to have his attention, but when he kept trying to swing me around in the crowded space, I advised him that his moves weren't really appropriate given the limited room. He pulled me into the bar area where there were fewer people, but still wasn't a great place for that type of dancing. In between talking, he started to kiss me. As I reveled in the feeling of being desired, I was initially open to seeing where it might lead, but soon realized that a) this Moroccan

French man was departing early in the morning to return home to France and b) he was already quite drunk. Neither was an appealing attribute and, as a combination were even less so, thus I bid him *bon voyage* and returned to the dance floor.

Later, as Gigi and I were getting water at the water station, a guy garbed in animal attire and lots of glitter asked if I was supposed to be a cheetah. With no specific species in mind when I designed my outfit, I replied that I was simply dressed in a generic cat print but asked him if he were playing some sort of animal bingo, looking to check off all the creatures on his list. (He wasn't.) We continued our banter and went to dance together.

I learned that his name was Christian, but our conversation was very un-Christian as we talked about group sex parties, turn-ons and similarly sexy topics. He had invited me to join him in the hot tub, but I declined, not wanting to get undressed or wet. We then found a quiet corner by ourselves to get more intimately acquainted. But I eventually excused myself to go to the restroom, and ultimately didn't return, since it was getting quite intense. It felt like things were escalating beyond kissing and caressing, and I knew that I didn't wish to accept his invitation to go back to his place. It was too much, too soon.

Back on the dance floor, a guy with bunny ears turned to me and demanded, "Dance with me!" I admonished him for not using the "magic word" (aka please). He remedied his error and I consented to dance with him. As we danced, he began to get closer and was then grinding against me. Intensely. At first, I thought it was a little sexy, but over time, I grew uncomfortable, not finding any pleasure in it, instead feeling merely like a receptacle for him.

I advised him that we could continue to dance together, but without all of the dick contact. He was very put out by my request and couldn't understand why I had changed my mind, so I left him on the dance floor. A part of me felt badly and questioned myself as to whether I had led him on, but logically I knew that I had every right to respect my own boundaries and ask him to do the same. A bit later, Gigi and I made arrangements to head home, but before we did, I ran into Christian again who gave me his number.

The next morning, I texted Christian so that he would have my number as well and we began an explicit discussion about threesomes and D/s (Domination/submission) power exchange (he claimed to be a Dominant). Despite the intensity of our encounter, I had enjoyed his company the night before and was intrigued by his potential Dom persona and the sexcapades that might ensue.

However, as the thread about threesomes shifted from a general discussion to a more specific request as to whether I had friends I could ask to participate, I told him we were getting ahead of ourselves and requested a date sans glitter to get to know each other first. There was no reply. At all. By mid-week, I was really annoyed at his blatant dismissal of me, so I carefully crafted a text message calling him out for his rude behavior. He immediately responded with an apology and I felt vindicated, hoping that he would consider improving his behavior with other women in the future.

Overall, I had enjoyed attending the party and felt that I had learned a lot about which experiences were pleasurable for me and which weren't. So, when another friend mentioned the August edition of House of Love, I thought it would be fun to return. This time the theme was Red, so I donned a red corset on top and a similar skirt/fishnets/heels combo below.

Gigi was again on-board, and this time Viktor was to be a part of the festivities. I was both excited and nervous to have Viktor in attendance as it would be our first foray together at this type of an event since our decision to pursue non-monogamy.

Before heading to House of Yes, we met up with Gigi and shared our general desires for the evening. While I wasn't sure what to expect this time compared to last time, I generally looked forward to another fun night of dancing and flirting. I also felt that I was getting clearer on what were turn-offs (overt grinding) and what were turn-ons (compliments and kisses). And admittedly, I hoped to run into

Christian to have my own *Pretty Woman* moment — Hi! Nice to see you. Remember when we talked about threesomes and you blew me off? Big mistake![4]

I wasn't sure how best to balance my desire to meet potential lovers with my desire to make sure that Viktor had a good time. In this regard, I was really glad that Gigi would be with us thinking that if we all danced together, it wouldn't hamper anyone's ability to attract attention and appear available, rather than if Viktor and I were dancing as a pair. In hindsight, I should have voiced these concerns with Viktor before we went and saved us some awkward moments, but this was new territory for both of us. And, despite a few hiccups, it generally went well, but more communication is never a bad thing.

Early on in the night, Gigi received a spanking from a leather-clad guy. Although she enjoyed the sensation play, she did joke that she might be a bit sore sitting down the next day. I briefly considered following her lead, but since Viktor and I had learned about such play during a D/s class a few years ago, I decided that there wasn't enough time or trust to calibrate the intensity preference at the party and chose to forgo the opportunity. But I did want to experience that kind of play under more conducive circumstances in the future.

Once her spanking was complete, we headed to the dance floor. Not long after, a guy started to dance with me and introduced himself as Andy. Soon Andy was teaching me ballroom dance moves (it was much less crowded this time due to the Labor Day holiday weekend). It was a lot of fun and I took great delight in the playfulness and connection. He offered to buy me a drink, and we headed outside to get to know one another. Among our topics of conversation, he asked me what my fetishes were (given that we were at a fetish party) and I shared that I was into bondage as a way to more fully surrender.

---

[4] In the film, Vivian says to the salesclerk, "I was in here yesterday. You wouldn't wait on me. You work on commission right? Big mistake. Big. Huge! I have to go shopping now."

A few moments later, as I was mid-sentence, Andy began to kiss me — his own way of (gently) forcing me to surrender. I felt into the kiss, decided that I liked it and kissed him back. We continued to kiss and talk for some time. Throughout our interaction, it was clear that he was very into me (or at least good at pretending he was), paying me beautiful compliments and calling me perfect. This was the type of attention that I craved: to be seen and to feel truly desired.

Andy wanted more privacy and took me to one of the single-stall bathrooms. He kissed me and then went down on me, but it wasn't relaxing or particularly pleasurable amidst the noise of partygoers banging on the door, so I stopped him, and we exited the bathroom. From there, we went to watch some bad '70s porn in the designated porn room. But eventually I grew bored with the movies and we returned to the dance floor. Upon our return, we coincidentally found Viktor who expressed his interest in spending time with me. I explained the situation to Andy who respectfully took his leave.

As I participated in these varied experiences with Andy, I kept checking in with myself to make sure that I was doing what was in my pleasure. I was trying to tease out what I was doing for me instead of doing things for men or doing them simply because they were expected. In theory, those days were over, but old habits die hard. And I was understanding how I wanted the attention and pursuit as it made me feel even sexier, added to my confidence and fed my turn-on.

I did find Andy again before we left and got his number, sending a quick text since he didn't have his phone on him. He texted the next day, following through on an invite he had issued the evening before but, as I had had a scant four hours of sleep (if that), I asked for a raincheck and spent the night at home with Viktor.

As is often the case with texting, my conversation with Andy left me unclear as to whether or not we had a date set for the Sunday afternoon after we had met at the party. Given the ambiguity (he had offered up the date, but had not finalized a time or place), I only semi-prepared to meet up with him (which meant no make-up and a mismatched bra and panty set) as I headed to my dance class wondering if I would hear from him or not.

About 30 minutes into my commute, Andy texted that he was looking forward to seeing me that afternoon. I confessed my confusion and asked if he had a specific plan in mind. After his overt sexual advances at the party, I was cautiously optimistic that he would suggest a real date and not just invite me over to his apartment to hook up. His suggestion that we meet for a bite, drink or whatever else we wanted made me feel better about his intentions and I left it to him to choose the venue although I did express a desire to be outside given the lovely weather.

Andy advised me to meet him at the Standard Hotel in the Meatpacking District. There is always that moment of fear as to whether or not you will recognize the person you met at a dark party, but we found each other on the sidewalk without incident.

Once we had said hello, we took the elevator up to the hotel's rooftop, which boasted spectacular views of New York City and the Hudson River. After we ordered cocktails, we scored a spot on the couch with a lovely waterfront vista and spent time sharing more about ourselves. We also talked about our interests in connection with dating each other as well as the particulars of my situation. As a single dad not wanting to get too entangled with someone, my open marriage status seemed to be a good fit for him.

During our conversation, Andy shared stories about some of his past dating experiences and revealed that he enjoyed having sex in situations or circumstances where there was the danger of being caught. Aha! I said, so you do have a fetish after all; you are an exhibitionist! He hesitantly agreed. (Now I understood the whole bathroom thing at House of Yes).

Every so often we would kiss, but I was uncomfortable to let the kisses linger too long since it was broad daylight and not an appropriate place for excessive public displays of affection. But, despite my slight discomfort, I did enjoy kissing him.

We had initially arrived on the rooftop in shade, but over time the sun had burned through the clouds, brightening the sky and heating up the day. The heat was welcome, but we were sweating quite a bit and eventually Andy suggested that we get up from our spot to take in another view.

I followed him down a flight of stairs, passed the bar and into the restroom area. Andy opened the door to one of the bathrooms, displaying not only the expected commode and sink, but also a floor-to-ceiling window overlooking The High Line. We were too high up to see any details, but the view was spectacular and there was definitely the feeling of being seen given all of the glass.

Andy drew me inside the stall with him, locked the door and began to kiss me in earnest. This was definitely well outside my comfort zone, but I decided to push my edges and allow the kisses to escalate. At least there was no one banging on the door this time.

Soon my skirt was pushed up and my panties were pulled down as Andy brought his mouth to my pussy and proceeded to taste me. I was nervous about getting in trouble, but, simultaneously, it felt thrilling to be with him in this manner. And, while I wasn't fully able to relax into his touch, it did feel really good and I felt very turned on.

I declined to return the favor orally for a variety of reasons and was certainly not ready to have intercourse with him since we still barely knew each other, but I did help pleasure him to climax, which he appreciated greatly. Andy had previously admitted to having masturbated twice since having met me on Friday and it was flattering and sexy to feel that I had generated such turn-on in someone.

After we cleaned up and departed the bathroom area, we sat on a couch and continued to talk for a while. Then we both had to head to our respective homes and Andy walked me to the subway, noting that he would like to see me again. It had truly been a delightful afternoon!

As the "Summer of Sexiness" was technically drawing to a close, I was still enjoying the journey as my sexual awakening continued to unfold. As Labor Day arrived, Viktor and I wanted one last hurrah before the pressures of work and life were permitted to press down on us once again. Well, maybe that was a bit too dramatic, but we did feel that it would be our last opportunity to head to the beach for the season. Thus, we were delighted when the day appeared to be a beautiful one, perfect for enjoying the sun and sand.

I had visited Gunnison Beach, the nude beach at New Jersey's Sandy Hook National Park, earlier in the summer with a friend and had had a really great time (my first time at a nude beach). Viktor was eager to experience it for himself, so our beach destination was easy, and we got ourselves ready, packing up the car with beach towels, sandwiches and beverages.

On the ride south, Viktor and I spent a lot of time talking about the Summer of Sexiness and how we were feeling about the various encounters that had occurred over the past four months. We also discussed our desires going forward, especially regarding date nights and "sex labs." We were both very much interested in exploring orgasm and pleasure without the goal of intercourse as a way to heighten our connection and expand our repertoire. It was a very cathartic and healing conversation as we opened up, expressed fears and spoke the truth. In a word, powerful! By the time we arrived in Sandy Hook we felt extremely connected to one another and ready for a fabulous day.

We set up our umbrella, beach blanket and towels and settled in for the day. It was hot — heat advisory hot — so we quickly divested of our clothing and hit the waves. It was glorious to float in the water *au naturelle*, enjoying the beauty and each other's company. After a while we were ready to return to our beach site, where we dried off, enjoyed our lunch and briefly napped. Later, we turned our attention to our Kindles, reveling in the chance to sit back, relax and read.

Suddenly, Viktor sat up, put down his book and exclaimed, "Isn't that Jake and Mia?" I looked over to where he was pointing and saw Mia in the distance. While I had mused that it would be cool to run into them at the beach earlier in the day, I hadn't really considered it to be a likely possibility given that a) we hadn't been in touch with them in several weeks, b) didn't know their holiday plans and c) it was a crowded beach! Yet here they were. Viktor ran after them lest we lose them in a sea of umbrellas and beach goers. They were delighted to see us and quickly invited us to come visit with them once they were settled.

Earlier in the month Jake had more explicitly expressed his interest in me, noting that the connection and chemistry that he and I shared was actually quite rare within the swingers' lifestyle. It meant a lot to receive these compliments and I shared that I felt blessed to have met him and Mia.

Viktor and I enjoyed frolicking on the beach and in the water with them that afternoon. At times Jake was very close to me, holding me close and kissing me. It felt exhilarating and vulnerable since we were naked and in public, but I welcomed the interaction. I was not sure that I was a swinger, but I did feel connected to Jake and Mia and was so happy to have them in Viktor's and my life.

Wanting to want

With the fall season upon us, I had learned so much about myself and my sexuality. In addition to my experiential exploits, I also spent time on self-reflection, trying to make sense of the past and present. I had focused a lot on the concept of desire but had also discovered that there was so much more to it. While I had initially thought that I was just seeking desire — the desire to have sex — as I proceeded in my sexploration, I felt certain that desire was actually enmeshed in turn-on and arousal, so it was challenging to tease out the individual strands of this issue for me.

In this regard, although I had begun this pursuit thinking that it was just a lack of desire — aka low libido — that was the root cause of my "problem." Yet, I now saw that it was much more layered and nuanced, and that libido was important, but insufficient.

Equally vital was the realization that desire (and eventually arousal) needed to stem from me. For years I had been under the mistaken belief that desire, and arousal were the (sole) result of sexual chemistry. I had wondered if the initial chemistry I had felt with Viktor all those years ago had simply vanished and thus severed our sexual connection, since I no longer seemed to feel that spark with him.

Instead, I finally understood that it was up to me to turn myself on, to determine what it was that lit me up, brought me pleasure and awakened my body in a sensual and sexual manner. I now knew that I couldn't rely on my partner to do it. If nothing else, it was unfair. But, more importantly, it wasn't a reasonable expectation.

However, it was fair (and helpful) to share my turn-ons with my partner once I had identified them. This was the stage I was at, in this moment, wanting to identify my turn-ons. I was trying to figure out: What was it that really ignited my desire and revved up my body to want to have sex (in any and all of its myriad forms)?

I was still struggling with these concepts and how they related specifically to me and my body. I no longer felt the shame associated with sex, but, having neglected this part of me for so long, it was hard to know where or how to begin to answer these questions.

In many ways, my body had been asleep for so long and I had fallen into bad habits as well, which made it difficult to understand what I was feeling, what I wanted and what I needed.

While my initial foray into dating those past few months definitely fed into my turn-on — the sexting, the attention and the newness of it all — most of it fell (and felt) flat once things proceeded into more overt territory. The inability to relax and surrender influenced things for sure, but I think a lot of it still hinged on my need to better understand just what it was that turned me on as well as on having a partner who cared (and wanted this information) and had the patience to provide me with whatever that turned out to be.

All of this brought me to a place of confusion, but also of hope. I knew that I needed to put in the time and effort to truly know myself in this context. I also knew that Viktor was as committed to this as much as I was, so, yes, I had hope that we would get to a place on the other side where sex and desire came more easily for me, leading to more frequent and better sex for us.

And, while finding my desire and turn-on could be a challenge in itself, there was another equally challenging piece to the puzzle: staying present. Although I was unaware that I was doing it, for years I would check out during sex. Yes, my body was physically there, but my mind was elsewhere. I was going through the motions, but I was not truly engaged or connected to Viktor. It wasn't until I read Madeleine Castellanos' book, *Wanting to Want*, that I became aware of my tendency to wander. I would literally zone out as if my mind and body were completely disconnected from one another.

Reading Madeleine's book late one night while Viktor was out of town on a business trip, I was suddenly struck by an intense sadness and began to sob loudly and uncontrollably. At first, I didn't know why I was so overcome with emotion, but I gradually recognized that I was mourning the loss of my sex life. Although I hadn't ever forgotten all of the various sexual misadventures that I had experienced early in life, it wasn't until that moment that I started to piece it together — seeing the thread that ran through all of them.

I realized that from the time I was a teen, I had been giving myself (my body) away to men in search of love and attention, but mistook their interest in me and instead, was left feeling used, abandoned, ashamed and dirty for putting myself into these situations. I also felt intense anger at myself for not finding my voice to honestly say what I did or didn't want in each particular situation. And even when I thought I was being a sexually empowered woman in college, I continued to give away my power in not asking for what I wanted and needed, putting the men's pleasure ahead (or more often instead) of mine. I repeated this pattern for years, oblivious that there even was a pattern, until I got married, but likely somewhere along the way I shut myself down to protect myself.

Now that I was conscious of my reaction, I was trying really hard to truly be present. I didn't want to have sex with Viktor (or anyone else) until I was clear with myself that I really *wanted* to be having sex. And, if I concluded that I didn't want to, then I promised myself that I would stop. If I decided that I did wish to continue having sex, I needed to focus on being in the moment — taking an active role and staying engaged with my partner.

This was difficult for me as I unlearned ingrained habits and overcame the negative experiences that caused me to adopt them in the first place. I knew that I had given myself sexually to men in the past for the wrong reasons. I was not going to find myself wrong for making those decisions (I'd done enough of that already), but I did want to recognize the toll those choices had taken on my sex life and identify ways to improve it going forward. I was healing, albeit slowly, learning to forgive myself and acknowledging that I now knew how to protect myself from, and (I hoped) prevent, these situations.

Part of the solution lay in appealing to my sensual blueprint (as per Miss Jaiya's Blueprints), allowing me to get out of my head and into my body. I had found that a relaxing, sensual massage could do wonders to put me more in the mood. Additionally, I had experimented with edibles because marijuana didn't interfere with your ability to orgasm the way alcohol did, but it did help quiet my mind and prohibit metacognition.

Moreover, I was trying to check in with myself. "Where were my thoughts at this moment?" I asked. "What was I thinking/ feeling/ doing during sex, bringing me back to myself and to my partner?"

In time, this would come more naturally, but for now I was rebuilding my neural pathways and creating more positive sexual experiences that would turn me on instead of pushing me to tune out.

In light of these recent musings, I soon had an opportunity to find out. Ever since our date at the Standard Hotel, Andy continued to text and occasionally telephone me. His texts and conversations were almost always overtly sexual and while I enjoyed the tantalizing nature of them, it was a bit intense for me to receive from someone I didn't know well.

As the months progressed, these interactions were happening within the context of the Kavanaugh trial and numerous Facebook posts from friends outing their attackers and generally describing their own sexual assaults. While I applauded their bravery in confronting the past, it was extremely triggering for me, reminding me of my own past. I sharply recalled those situations in which I had allowed myself to be used or taken advantage of sexually, which further heightened my concerns (and instilled a bit of a flight reflex) when it came to Andy.

In an effort to clearly manage expectations, I continually let him know that although I was interested in being intimate with him, I was not yet ready to engage in sexual intercourse. He referred to these expectations as my "rules," which ruffled me a bit. However, since he assured me that he understood my intentions, I was confident that we were on the same page, even if his reference to them seemed a bit dismissive. But, in hindsight, I should have seen it as a red flag.

After numerous texts and phone calls, Andy finally proceeded to make plans with me. An avid roller-disco dancer, he invited me to join him at an event that coming Friday. He advised that he already had his ticket (and his own skates) and that I would need to purchase a ticket and skate rental. Since the event started at 6:00 p.m., I asked him what time he planned to arrive. He responded that he would be there between 7:30 and 8:00 p.m., after tending to his kids. While I respected his need to take care of his children, a 30-minute window was a bit large when arranging to meet someone...on a date!

The more I engaged in these interactions, it became clearer that my intuition was spot on. If I felt that something might be off; it was. Full stop.

It didn't feel right, but I decided to take a chance and say yes to the unusual plans. The ticket price itself wasn't very expensive and I thought it might be fun. But, when I proceeded to purchase my ticket, I discovered that there were no more skate rentals available. I knew that he already had his ticket in hand and was committed to going, so I made alternate plans for Friday night. But now that I had experienced his planning approach, I knew I needed to be upfront about what I wanted and needed from him.

I texted him the next morning,

"I had been looking forward to seeing you on Friday, but after we hung up the phone, I looked into the tickets at the Roller Disco event and discovered that the skate rental tickets were sold out. Since you said that you already had your tickets, I have now made other plans for Friday evening. Sorry to miss you, but frankly this particular plan did not feel like a real date and I should have spoken up at the time. If you would like to try again to meet up, I would kindly ask that you make an actual plan for us rather than leaving me to fend for myself and then meet you somewhere at an approximate time."

Andy immediately texted back three emojis of hands waving goodbye. Clearly, he wasn't up to treating me with the care and consideration I wanted and deserved. Admittedly, his quick dismissal of me stung, but I truly knew that it wasn't a good fit between us and that he couldn't (or at least, wouldn't) provide me with the level of respect and attention I desired. I knew I deserved so much more.

Meanwhile, since Hank and I had left things on a friendly note, I had reached out to him at the start of the school year (he was a teacher) and wished him all the best for the new semester. Among our conversation, he noted: "Hope you are well. If you are open to hanging out, I am down."

Thinking that we might remain friends (he's generally a nice person), I responded favorably, advised him that I would follow up after my vacation, and a few weeks later, asked if he wanted to meet me at a wine bar near his apartment. He consented and we made plans. However, on the Saturday before our Monday night meeting, he cancelled, citing his wish to find a girlfriend. I was very confused since I thought we were merely meeting as friends, but I guess I had been mistaken. (At least in my book, men can have female friends and still try to find a girlfriend.)

So, I said, "Sayonara," to Hank, again. But we clearly didn't communicate well, so it was all for the best. It was just another opportunity to permit myself to get clarity on what I did and didn't want as well as determine what behavior I found acceptable or unacceptable.

Eyes wide open

By the end of October, I had decided that the Summer of Sexiness was still firmly with us; it wasn't a season, but rather, a state of mind. Thus, with its theme of All Hallows Eve and a mandate to don masks, I headed to a third erotic party, this time with Viktor in tow. The hostess further suggested more formal attire than she had previously done, which imbued the event with an Eyes Wide Shut vibe. And, as an added dimension, she underscored the importance of being unmasked, revealing what lay beneath and exposing what was hidden from others.

Also, this was my first time attending a play party with Viktor (the two previous ones I had attended without him) and with my friend, Dan. Their attendance added both excitement and anxiety as I considered their needs as well as my own.

After talking Dan off the figurative ledge a few times (his last text on his way to the party read, "Should be there 10:45. Don't take it personally if I leave at 10:50," and included a "scream" emoji), I left his actual experience up to fate. But, the day before the party, Viktor and I spent considerable time talking about our desires, expectations and plans for our joint attendance. To a certain extent, we wanted to be sure we went into the experience with eyes wide open.

We decided that we would clearly acknowledge our marital bond to those we met and that I would be less focused on finding someone, placing the evening's emphasis on Viktor instead of me. Since I had participated in more adventures during the past six months than Viktor had, I knew that Viktor harbored a slight envy at that lack and was happy to step back this time. Further, while we had attended the House of Love party together during Labor Day weekend, he had left that party with mixed emotions about it.

After we talked through those feelings, he felt much better and became clearer about his own desires and intentions for this event. In particular, he wanted to find someone to kiss during the evening (and asked for my assistance as a wing woman to make that happen) and he also hoped to find a woman who might be interested in a sexual liaison with the two of us.

On party night, I took the theme to heart, carefully layering a black bodysuit, with a suspender harness under my chiffon, bead-embellished gown, along with fishnet stockings, stiletto heels and an intricate black mask. I was unsure how much I would reveal during the night and enjoyed the idea of being more covered up than I had at the previous events. I also liked knowing that while I looked good in my dress, I held a sexy secret underneath.

Upon arrival at the venue, I introduced Viktor to the hosts and was then promptly greeted by Hank (more warmly than expected). The two finally met, which was less awkward that I had anticipated. We headed out into the backyard and soon found Dan, sitting by the fire pit, along with some other friends of ours.

As we stood outside chatting, the autumn air was crisp, with a slight chill, but the space was buzzing with anticipation as the guests eagerly awaited the opening ritual. At the appointed moment, an amazing ballet burlesque performer kicked off the celebration, which was followed by an intimate pussy worship ceremony and concluded with a sex magic spell. We were then released to play.

Soon after our arrival, Viktor met Marni with whom he really clicked. At first, I felt a little wary of the attention he was giving to her, but as I examined those feelings, I realized that it wasn't jealousy per se, but rather, an unwillingness to share my toys. However, once I saw how happy Viktor was in spending time with her, I felt really good about it. As Dan noted correctly (so obviously pleased with himself to have a perfect occasion on which to use the term): compersion. Any negativity or insecurity melted away and I was simply free to enjoy the experience.

Once again, the erotic party provided an opportunity to explore a variety of sensual experiences including erotic massage, flogging and Shibari bondage rope. I briefly considered getting tied up as an interesting comparison to the Shibari experience that Viktor had engaged in with me for my birthday earlier that month but decided that I was really more interested in impact play.

After we introduced ourselves, the resident flogger gave me a general introduction to flogging as well as an overview of what to expect during the session. I was extremely impressed with his professionalism in addition to his DIY skills, having made many of the floggers himself, from a combination of household items, including a Swiffer handle. After the "orientation," I slipped off my dress and mask, revealing my lingerie, which he admired appreciatively. I straddled the flogging bench and waited for the first stroke.

While I didn't think that I had had a sexual response to the flogging, I did enjoy the experience, as the flogger demonstrated the differences in intensity and sensation with each flogger type; some of the hits were gentler as they landed on my exposed ass, while others were more intense in their sting (what I later learned was referred to as thuddy and stingy). Afterward, the residual heat and pain lingered in an exquisite way. I was definitely interested in exploring impact play more in the future.

Prior to the flogging session, I had been standing in the sensual play area with Dan, observing others as they participated in these options. He expressed an interest in leaving soon but decided to stay to watch my flogging session. Near the end of the session, Viktor arrived with Marni, catching a glimpse of the final swats before I got up from the bench.

At that point, Dan was sated from the experience and I kissed him goodbye as he headed out. I then went back outside, where I reconnected with Tim, who I had met at the previous two parties. Afterward, I joined Viktor and Marni at the firepit, enjoying spending time with them both. Marni decided that she wanted to experience flogging, too, so the three of us returned inside, as Viktor and I sat together watching Marni's session. Feeling both satiated and sleepy, Viktor requested a car to take us home, as he exchanged phone numbers with Marni, in anticipation of a future date for the three of us. He had manifested all of his desires!

The seasonality of sex

Like the seasons and the moon, our lives are cyclical. We wax and wane. There is growth and death, repeating itself time and time again.

There is a warmth during the Summer fueled by the sun, which nourishes us and allows us to expand. Come Winter, days become darker and shorter, providing us with a time to reflect and stand still.

In this vein, the launch of the "Summer of Sexiness" in May of 2018 marked a huge expansion for me. I pressed edges, determined my boundaries, experimented and experienced so much. I felt energized and alive during all of my adventures and explorations.

But, as autumn came and went, I began to feel lethargic and less interested in sex. My desire had waned significantly, and I wondered if I was done. Then, as I got ready to welcome the Winter Solstice, I was reminded that there was nothing wrong with the need to go inward for a time after such a sustained period of growth.

I was learning to listen to my body and to honor what she was feeling in all seasons. I recognized that I was in a period of contraction and was choosing to find myself right instead of worrying about how that might be wrong. I honored my need to rest and recharge, while at the same time I reaffirmed my commitment to this journey.

Also, as the new year dawned, I took the opportunity to reflect once again on what I wanted, needed and desired. I saw that it was important to me to maintain a deep connection with Viktor. And to do so, we needed to redouble our efforts to schedule date nights and make specific plans that brought us together on a regular basis.

I needed to re-establish my Yoni egg practice since I wanted to enhance my sensitivity and ability. I needed to recommit to self-pleasure and to explore and practice what I had learned from Sheri Winston's book, *Anatomy of Female Arousal.*

I also needed to get clarity on what I wanted with regard to dating, sex and intimacy. In this regard, I was still unclear. I liked the idea of dating, but so far, none of those experiences have been satisfying in the way I had hoped they would.

I had had both positive and negative experiences in the bedroom, all of which had been learning experiences as I learned about my turn-on and took responsibility for my desire and orgasm.

And, I had learned to trust myself and set firm boundaries. I would no longer do anything that my body was not wholeheartedly on board with. I would protect myself and my body. It felt so good to have come this far. And, yet there was much more to investigate, so much further to go.

With the Solstice behind us, I knew that the days were slowly getting longer and brighter and had no doubt that a new season of expansion was on the horizon. But until then I honored my need to renew and recharge so that I would be ready when the time came.

Adventures in online dating

As winter carried on, Viktor and I signed up for a (new to us) dating app especially geared for non-conventional relationships called Feeld. Initially, Viktor took the lead in identifying potential matches, focused on finding a guy to bring into our bedroom and met at least two of them in person. This triggered me a bit since such actions made things more real and tangible and I had a few moments of (mild) panic. But I was not sure precisely where the fear came from. What was I afraid of?

With this recent emphasis on plurality, I pushed myself to examine what I wanted. I also felt that I needed to take ownership of this process and thus became active on the app as well, matching with a few couples. Yet nearly each time, I freaked out and clicked "later" instead of "chat now."

Having briefly dated this past summer and fall, I noticed that, with dating, I felt wanted, adored and cared for (when it was done right, i.e., more like Dan than like Hank). I enjoyed being the center of attention as well as the newness and discovery and the mystery of getting to know someone one.

But, frankly, I was confused as to what I wanted with regard to threesomes and foursomes. I craved more connection than those experiences would provide. Moreover, I knew that I wanted to be pursued. I liked that piece of dating; being wanted enough for someone to make an effort. That was not to say that Viktor didn't make an effort; he truly did, but I hungered for more. However, I did feel guilty for wanting this, because it seemed like I should be able to get what I needed from Viktor alone.

Dating also seemed less scary in one way because it felt more like a slow dance of getting to know someone while the threesome/foursome approach seemed much more focused on sexcapades. Finding singles for threesomes (or couples for foursomes) on an app felt scary and contrived and I worried that by matching with them I was promising something — aka sex — and I was not sure I was ready for that at the outset.

Yet, part of me wanted to feel the cavalier freedom to hop from bed to bed, but the rest of me feared having to deliver, and I worried about being able to relax and surrender with these people who I had never met. Plus, having never used a dating app before, I wondered about the idea of meeting someone online and whether I would feel any chemistry once I actually met them in person.

Of course, logically I knew that I was not signing on any dotted line or promising anything simply by chatting online, but the anxiety, while short-lived, was real.

Not long after our initial foray into online dating, I decided to jump into the deep end with both feet. I started clicking on a few profiles on the dating app and before I knew it (once I got over the initial panic of matching), I was engaged in several different conversations.

I had mostly selected single men. Not because I had specifically made the choice of "single" over "plural," but more because I felt that Viktor had the plural route covered with the connections he was making on the app.

Having never done online dating before, the concept was foreign, yet intriguing as I read through a wide variety of profiles. Mostly, I wanted to mix and match my preferred faces with the more alluring descriptions, but I did find a few that held my visual and intellectual interest. I tried to match personal interests (yes to wine) with sexual predilections (no to anal) and soon had two dates scheduled the following week.

I was still skeptical about meeting someone in person that I had only previously seen online, but the only way to find out was to go ahead, so I did.

My first date was with Jon. He hadn't listed much in his profile, but I was very attracted to his photos and looked forward to meeting him.

I was a little nervous in anticipation of his arrival, but since I had no real attachment to the outcome at that point, it was simply pleasure research. Mostly, I was excited.

I arrived at the venue first and texted Jon that I was seated at the bar wearing a striped dress. He easily found me and said hello. Our initial greeting was a bit awkward, as we briefly hugged and finally revealed our actual names (we had been using pseudonyms on the app) to each other. But we were soon at ease with one another, being flirty, open and comfortable sharing on a range of topics.

At one point, he leaned in closer and we gently kissed. I was definitely turned on and was sorry it was over so soon. A while later, Jon picked up the check and we walked out together, saying goodbye at the corner with another kiss.

The next morning, I saw a sweet text from him that he had sent the night before. I replied and after a few messages back and forth, he said he would love to see me again. Swoon! I readily agreed and we made a date for a few weeks hence.

I tried not to think about him too much, but there was an instant attraction and I thought there could be real potential for a long-term lover situation, which was something that I felt that I really desired.

In the meantime, I made a date with another guy for later that week, one with a guy and his girlfriend for the following week and had a few chats going on in the app with some other people. Again, it was additional pleasure research as well as an entry into defensive dating.

One thing that I had noticed was that I craved attention. I loved the adoration I felt when I matched with someone and then got a text from that stranger, which was further heightened when the text included compliments about me.

At the time, I took note of how these different interactions made me feel and tried to stay grounded and realistic. But, if nothing else, there was no doubt that after my season of contraction, I was back. A brief discussion with a friend revealed a similar re-awakening and we both wondered if the Chinese New Year, with its lunar, more feminine wave was, at least partly, to blame.

The Friday after my date with Jon, I met up with Patrick who I had also met on the app. Patrick suggested that we meet at one of his favorite Italian restaurants, which turned out to be a cute, neighborhood place with good food and great service.

Patrick had arrived ahead of me (I appreciated his punctuality) and after a few minutes of confusion, we found each other, and he warmly welcomed me. He had gotten himself a ginger-flavored cocktail and advised me that the restaurant grated its own ginger. Then, he offered me a taste of his and I was sold. We were then whisked away to our table and immediately tumbled into various conversations. In fact, we got so engrossed in conversation that we had to force ourselves to take a break and look at the menu before the waiter returned yet another time to take our order. ·

Once our orders had been placed, we renewed our discussions, flowing fluidly from one topic to another, finding synergies in our current lives and relationships and otherwise connecting to one another. We also shared past experiences and adventures within the sex community and our own journeys.

After dinner, Patrick offered to hail us a taxi and drop me off at my apartment on his way home (he lived in the neighborhood adjacent to mine) and we continued talking as we walked out into the street, but now started kissing as well. The kisses persisted throughout the cab ride and were a lot of fun. I was definitely glad that I had met him.

Before the date, I had told Viktor that I planned to come home relatively early (anticipating being home by 9:30 from my 7:00 p.m. date) and have sex with him. Unfortunately, I lost track of time and came home much later than I had promised. In fact, I had never thought to check the clock and didn't know it was just a few minutes before midnight until I walked in the door to Viktor's (understandable and justified) anger.

I owned my faults and sincerely apologized to him. I realized that I hadn't treated him with the respect he deserved, and I felt really terrible about hurting him. We had a very reasonable discussion about his hurt feelings, and he heard my apology. We were able to really listen to each other without raising voices or exacerbating the situation. We both also realized that my error was unrelated to being out on a date and could just have easily happened if I had been out with friends. It wasn't the first time something like this had happened.

Somewhat seriously, somewhat in jest, Viktor demanded that I make it up to him by undressing him and having the sex I promised. He made it clear that I had to do all the work and also noted that he didn't want me to simply apply some lube and make it a quickie. I was in agreement with my "punishment" and slowly untied his pajama bottoms with my mouth and then gently tugged them down and off. I removed my bra and panties and straddled him, sliding his shaft up and down along my slit, beginning to get aroused and wet. Viktor next requested a blowjob and I readily complied, doing my best to over-deliver on his expectations and presumably did since he was quite hard and dripping when I resumed straddling him.

After a few minutes, I took him inside me and experienced intense orgasmic sensations, which pleasantly surprised me since there had been relatively minimal foreplay. Eventually Viktor climaxed, but, while it had felt really good to me, I still wanted to have an orgasm, since I hadn't really finished during intercourse.

I used my vibrator to satisfaction, culminating in an intense orgasm and then got up. A moment later, I started squirting (for the first time). Unfortunately, it coincided with a heavy menstrual cycle (which had seemed to have ceased when I had taken off my panties prior to sex) and suddenly there was blood squirting everywhere — on me, on the floor, on the sheets and eventually on the mattress pad and mattress.

It was both glorious and gross all at once. And the beauty was that instead of getting upset, Viktor simply called for me to grab a towel to begin cleaning everything up as quickly as possible. He made sure not to shame me or make me feel badly about the blood or mess and was really adamant about me not negating the experience of squirting.

After we had cleaned up, changed the sheets and gotten into bed, I shared my gratitude with him, reminded all over again how much I loved him.

In the days that followed, I had a flurry of texts from my myriad of admirers, including one from Patrick noting that he was taking the day off on Tuesday and asked if I would like to meet up for coffee or lunch. We arranged to meet at 1:00 p.m. after my dance class. At the last minute, we discovered that our chosen restaurant wouldn't be open in time, so we made a game-time decision to go to my favorite, local wine bar. I had mentioned the bar to Patrick on our first date, but he hadn't yet been.

I arrived a few minutes late and found Patrick at the bar, talking to the wine bar's owner, Bill. It turned out that the two of them knew each other from the past (more synchronicity). I greeted Patrick warmly but was admittedly anxious about being too demonstrative since Bill knew me and Viktor. I knew that I had to say something, or I would feel entirely stifled during our date.

So, I took a deep breath, walked over to the bar and told Bill I needed to tell him something. I asked him if he remembered making a cute comment on my Instagram account about polyamory in wine bars, a few months back. He didn't quite remember, but I left the "p word" hanging there to indicate what was presently going on. I wanted him to know that I wasn't cheating on Viktor and he didn't have to report me to the marriage police.

It was still a little awkward and embarrassing, mostly because there was only one other customer there (it was more a wine bar than lunch place), and it was brightly lit. Yet, I managed to focus on Patrick instead and we proceeded to have a lovely date.

We eventually agreed it was time to depart, so we left the wine bar, hugged and kissed for a few minutes on the sidewalk and then headed to our respective homes.

On a Tuesday night, Jon texted me: "Ice Cream? Wednesday or Friday?" I was excited to see his interest in seeing me again so soon, especially since we already had a date scheduled for Monday. Unfortunately, we realized that to make an ice cream meeting happen, we would need to twist ourselves into pretzels, so we abandoned the idea.

When I asked him if we were confirmed for Monday, he replied, yes. I then asked for details on the time and place because we had not discussed anything other than that it would be a daytime date on Monday. He texted back, "Menu: (wine emoji), (cheese emoji), followed by an address." Then, when I asked him what time I should arrive, he said we had from 10:00 a.m. to 6:00 p.m. It was so fucking hot!

A while later, he sent an image of his STI test results (indicating that he was sexually healthy). He admitted that it wasn't romantic, but he thought I would like to know. It was very much appreciated and added to my sense of trust and esteem of him. His actions were such a polar opposite to my dates from the summer and it was not only refreshing, but extremely welcome. I was very intrigued for Monday and tried to manage my expectations so that I would not be disappointed or overly expectant.

Meanwhile, my date (or rather, more of an initial meet and greet) with the couple, Josh and Lee, was lovely, though not particularly eventful. We met at a casual bar in Lee's neighborhood and spent two hours getting to know one another. I had found them on the app and had enjoyed my text exchanges with Josh. When we first matched, he had asked if I wanted to meet him on his own or with Lee. I replied that I was game to meet them both and explore whether or not we all clicked in person.

During our evening together, we covered a range of topics from careers, travel and pets to our experiences with the app, open relationships and sexual preferences. At the end of the evening, Josh asked me what I thought, and I expressed my interest in seeing them again. They invited me to return with them to Lee's apartment, but I politely declined, noting that I would savor the anticipation for when we did get together.

The next day I woke to a beautiful message from Josh...

"Hope you got home OK. So, upon discussing you/our evening afterwards (hope your ears weren't burning too badly) we came to a couple of conclusions: we both agree that you're stunning and can't wait to see you (and perhaps more of you) next, we're realizing were pretty sapiosexual or cultursexual or just plain ol' interesting-people-sexual. It's not that we don't find other people attractive or that we need the sapio-ness to be attracted to someone, but rather that you check ALL the boxes. And you're super sweet. Just thought I'd share. Night night!"

All of this seduction and flattery could go to a girl's head, but I wasn't complaining. Could all of this undo decades of self-doubt and judgment? Honestly it just could.

Love, sex and magick

For our Valentine's Day celebration, we decidedly chose to focus on just Jeannie and Viktor, not Jeannie, Viktor and someone else. We booked a room at the Essex House, which was the hotel where we had spent our wedding night. I even brought a copy of the original room receipt to share with the staff at check-in.

We were given a beautiful room with a view of Central Park and then took some time setting everything up — creating a makeshift pantry for our snacks and kicking off the weekend with a glass of Champagne. I had purchased a new set of Agent Provocateur lingerie for the occasion because I am a lingerie addict and also to imbue our new credit card with good vibes as this was the first purchase made on it.

Once we were ready, Viktor surprised me with a magical love spell that truly set the container for our celebration and created the perfect mood separating the week from the weekend and the mundane from the sacred.

We slowly turned our attention to each other with kisses and caresses. Then, Viktor really surprised me! He brought me to orgasm with Tantric energy breath without touching my genitals at all. I had no idea this was even possible. The only other somewhat similar experience I had had was when I had used Layla Martin's breathwork audio recording, using only my breath and energy flow to bring me to orgasm, but that had required a lot of focus from me. In this case, it was Viktor's focus on me. Wow! Afterwards, I continued to feel waves of orgasm come upon me throughout the evening, almost like aftershocks from an earthquake. It was an exquisite experience.

Throughout our time in the hotel, we simply enjoyed one another through touch and taste, indulging in delicious foods, titillating movies (a big thumbs up for Erica Lust's "Confessions" series) and much love. It was a reminder how important (and fun) it was to have the luxury of time to spend with your partner relishing in their company, their body and your shared intimacy.

A few days after Valentine's Day, I had my date with Jon. Unlike when I Googled "What to wear to a threesome," or, later, "What to wear to a foursome" (equally unhelpful), Googling "What to wear to a sex date," offered up numerous articles on the subject. For the most part, these articles recommended the avoidance of overly complex underwear, tricky clothing closures and heavy makeup.

In arranging our sex date, I had asked Jon for his preference among black, navy, pink and purple. He chose purple, so the lingerie choice was made. I then decided on thigh-high black stockings (sexy and easier than tights), a black leather skirt with a big zipper running down the back (quite easy to unzip and remove) and a velvet top (who doesn't love touching velvet?). Unfortunately, since the light in the room was harsh, we kept the lights off, so the lingerie big reveal was less revealing, but he still appreciated the bra and panties (and me!).

Just prior to my arrival, Jon texted me the room number and I went directly upstairs and knocked on the door. As much as I had been looking forward to our date, I was equally nervous since we had only had one previous (relatively short) date. However, after about 20 minutes or so, I felt reasonably relaxed as we started to talk, sip some wine and began to kiss. Since we had the whole day, we were able to take our time and not feel rushed to have sex.

He was very giving and patient and I found myself able to truly enjoy being with him. He initially went down on me and I surrendered enough to have an orgasm; not the most intense one, but I was pleasantly surprised it had happened at all, after my experiences with Hank and Kevin. We then engaged in 69, which I also enjoyed, especially in being able to give pleasure to him.

Actual intercourse was a bit more complicated because he was not used to condoms and had some difficulty with his erection, but we did manage to connect eventually. But again, I was really delighted with how easy it all seemed given our limited knowledge of one another and how new this still was to me. As it was, Jon was only the second man with whom I had had intercourse since this all began aside from Jake.

As we lay in bed, we drifted between verbal intimacy and physical intimacy, with Jon bringing me to orgasm several times throughout the afternoon. We also listened to music and shared fantasies and fetishes. He expressed interest in being spanked and trusted me to spank him since I had learned some techniques in a D/s class in the past. After I stopped spanking him, I asked him what he thought, and he revealed that he had an erection (score one for Jeannie). In return, when asked and admitted that I had not had my nipples bitten, Jon happily obliged, ultimately bringing me to orgasm (score one for Jon).

Eventually, it was nearly time to go, so we took a brief, sudsy shower together before gathering our things and heading out. Among our various conversations, I expressed how sexy I thought his invitation was and explained that if it hadn't been so sexy, I likely would have declined due to the newness of our relationship. In the spirit of full disclosure, Jon revealed that he had Googled, "How to ask for a sex date" (score one for Google).

The big "O"

As I struggled with understanding my own body and its ability to surrender sexually, orgasm continued to be on my mind. Defined by Wikipedia as a "discharge of sexual excitement," (so not a sexy definition), the big O, as in Orgasm, seemed to be a topic that was possibly very misunderstood by both men and women. And a video by Sex Educator, Layla Martin, focused on why 46% of women had difficulty with achieving orgasm, so it seemed to be on a lot of other people's minds as well.

As I typed that sentence, it struck me that the language we use can complicate things still further...Achieve! Really, it's not enough to simply *have* an orgasm, we have to *achieve* it! (And, interestingly, I unconsciously put that word in there; when I went to check the actual title for Layla's video it read: "This is why 46% of women *struggle* to orgasm").

Plus, if you Google the word orgasm, you get 490,000,000 hits, including results such as "How Many Types of Orgasm Am I Capable Of? (Hint: 14)" So, we now have 14 ways we are (or are not) achieving in this regard. Good grief! This was not to diminish the existence or value of the diversity of orgasms, but rather to underscore the extra burden of expectation that some might feel.

Consequently, there was so much pressure to perform and on top of that, it takes a woman much longer to get fully aroused. Yet, what messages do Hollywood, porn and others send us? Scenes in which the woman climaxes almost as soon as she is penetrated. Not to mention how quickly she is ready for penetration (as if), pushing us to presume that there must be something wrong with us or our bodies if we don't respond similarly. And, as Layla explained, this was compounded by years of shame and similarly negative messages around our sexuality. In a word, we were not supposed to be sexual unless we were whores.

So, with all of this swirling in our heads, how were we supposed to allow ourselves to relax, surrender and truly let go? To let go of judgment, of self-consciousness, of doubt, of body shame, all of it. How do we banish our anxiety that we are taking too long, are too loud, too demanding or all of the above?

The more I examined my own climax, I realized that there was no one answer, but rather we needed time, we needed trust, and we needed truth. We needed to feel truly desired. We needed to feel better about ourselves and our bodies. We needed to feel safe and comfortable to give feedback to our partner and, to do that, we needed knowledge of what turned us on and what turned us off and, equally important, general knowledge of our bodies (see Sheri Winston's book[5].

Moreover, having just returned from my tryst with Jon during which I was pleasantly surprised at how my body responded to his, I thought that practice might be critical, too. It may be that we needed to continually awaken our bodies with pleasure in order to fully experience it. And, while I was still not experiencing earth-shattering orgasms with my partners[6], I was finding that I was experiencing more pleasure during intercourse and that my body was discovering new ways to orgasm (though not quite 14, yet). It may sound funny, but I had never really understood what the big deal was about sex (read penetration) for so long. I was finally starting to get it.

Three weeks to the day of our first meeting, Patrick and I had our first intimate encounter. Given the close connection we had had since that initial five-hour date, I was very much looking forward to what would happen between us. I was not disappointed.

---

[5] Winston, Sheri. *Anatomy of Female Arousal.* 2010

[6] These seem to be generally reserved for my vibrator.

We met for a lovely dinner in the neighborhood and then headed to my apartment for "dessert." I briefly gave him a tour, opened a bottle of wine and then we moved to the guest room, shutting out the dog and the world. Over the next several hours we proceeded to delight in each other's bodies through oral and penetrative sex. My body was comfortable and relaxed in his presence as well as very turned on.

Later, we held each other, and I actually dozed off for a while — a rare occurrence for me. Energy renewed; we resumed our physical intimacy. Eventually, it was late (3:30 a.m.) and Patrick decided that he should head home, so I kissed him goodbye and reluctantly let him leave.

Nights of twine and poses

I initially encountered Ryan at the first erotic party I attended in May. As the Shibari master, Ryan introduced party guests to this Japanese sensual art, binding them with rope. But, aside from my curiosity about Shibari, I didn't give him a second thought. Afterwards, I had a slight pang of regret at not participating and resolved to do so at the next party, but, then chose not to spend the night waiting on the lengthy line (and ended up meeting Jake and Mia instead), so our paths still didn't cross.

At the third party, Viktor met Ryan when Ryan tied up Marni and they had had a brief discussion on their shared interest in Shibari, but I wasn't involved in those interactions. Thus, it wasn't until my fourth party that I was introduced to Ryan officially. He had become friends with Jason and Bettie, with whom we had connected before (and then met at) the party, and the five of us ended up hanging out around the fire pit.

As Ryan and I talked, I began to feel some chemistry and was very intrigued by him. Then, toward the end of the party, I had the exquisite pleasure of being bound and suspended by Ryan. I was definitely smitten but figured I wouldn't see him again until the next party. Fortunately, I was wrong.

A few days after the party, I received a Direct Message on Instagram from Ryan complimenting me on my erotic dance (I had been a part of the opening ritual at the party) and asking if he could see me again in the future. Butterflies! I immediately consented and he sent me his phone number. After several text exchanges, we tried to meet up late one night (Ryan's work schedule was not 9-5), but he kept getting held up at work. I eventually decided that it was too late to meet up but suggested that we talk on the phone as he drove home that night. It was a pleasure to speak with him and get to know him better.

As I planned dates with others, my mind kept traveling back to Ryan. I desired for him to ask me out but knew that his schedule was challenging and didn't want to hope for too much. However, at one point, I did let him know that I would be available on a particular Friday night (in case it was of interest to him, lol!).

At first, he responded that it was too far ahead to commit due to work, but he later reached out and invited me to join him at a pool party. I was excited about the event and seeing him but wasn't sure what to expect. It was better than I could have imagined.

Soon after we arrived, we stripped down to our bathing suits, checked our clothing and coats, and headed to the bar for drinks. We sat talking and soon started kissing. Ryan asked for general consent for the night, which I eagerly granted. Next, we headed into the pool, continuing to talk and kiss. As our kissing grew more intense, Ryan's fingers began to wander, traveling to my breasts and then, later, to my pussy. It was incredibly intimate for a public, well-lit event, but somehow the crowd seemed to fade, then disappear, and I was all but lost to everything but Ryan and his touch. Sigh!

After the party, we went out to a diner with his friends, splitting an order of blueberry pancakes and generally enjoying each other's company. By then, it was 2:30 a.m., but I knew that Viktor was still out at a rave and Ryan was happy to come home with me. I gave him a brief tour of the apartment that ended with the guest room, where we promptly disrobed and fell into bed, hungry to explore each other further, without the distraction of water and people. We chose to defer intercourse since it was late, but we shared the bliss of oral sex.

We continued to kiss, touch and talk, when, several hours later, we heard the apartment door open, indicating that Viktor had arrived home. Then there was a knock on the guest room door. I froze for a moment, but ultimately Ryan invited Viktor to come in. After we all chatted for a few minutes, at our urging, Viktor quickly undressed and climbed into bed with us. He began to tell us about his evening and we briefly shared about the pool party. Then we stopped talking and Ryan started to give Viktor a blowjob. Afterward, Viktor happily returned the favor.

Eventually they remembered about me (just kidding), and we all actively engaged in a magnificent threesome. It was amazing! It was incredibly erotic to watch Viktor and Ryan together and then receive their joint attention. I enjoyed the experience even more than my threesome with Jake and Mia. We all really clicked, and the chemistry seemed to abound on all sides — win-win-win for everybody! By 6:30 a.m., Ryan had to head home, and Viktor and I drifted off to sleep for a few hours, ecstatically content.

A few days after our first date, Ryan came over after work to spend the night with me. Viktor was out of town on business, so he wouldn't hijack our date this time around and it gave us a chance to really get to know each other better and explore our intimacy further.

Upon Ryan's arrival, I opened up a bottle of wine so we could relax into the evening and unwind from the day. It felt great to see him and be held and kissed.

I had dressed in a short plaid skirt, with garters and stockings underneath and wore tall, black boots since he had expressed interest in this type of look on our previous date. After we had enjoyed the wine and talked for a while, I asked him if he preferred to undress me himself or if he would like me to dance for him. He chose the latter, so I put on a song I had recently danced to in S Factor and proceeded to move for him. By the conclusion of the song, I had stripped off my top. We renewed our kissing as he pulled me onto his lap and removed my bra.

A while later, Ryan asked if I wanted to be tied up. I readily consented and he surprised me. Instead of taking me into the guest room, he guided me to stand in front of our Barcelona chair. He bound my arms behind my back, making sure that I was comfortable. He then wound the rope around my torso above my breasts, then below. I loved the deliberate and slow careful attention as he unfurled his hanks of rope and then applied his art to my body.

Once he was satisfied with my upper binding, he sat me down on the chair and gently reached for my left leg. He bent my leg and placed my foot on the chair before circling my ankle with the twine. I thought that he would bind my leg to itself as Viktor had previously done, but instead he pulled it straight and wide. I was thankful for my flexibility class and the sexiness of my stockings. Ryan then secured the rope to the back of the chair.

He repeated his ministrations on my right leg until I had both legs splayed open in front of me, held up by the ropes. I felt very provocative in this position as well as vulnerable, but I trusted and felt safe with Ryan. I tried to tune out everything and quiet my mind and did a reasonably good job considering that this was always a challenge for me.

He had teased me a bit during the set up, but now he turned his full attention to my pussy and breasts, turning me on slowly, then more intensely. His fingers slid along my underwear, then underneath as I gasped more audibly with each stroke. I felt how wet I was. Then, he tugged the panties down and began to taste me, bringing me higher and higher.

Afterwards, he took his time to remove the ropes, first releasing my legs and then freeing my arms. Next, he pulled me into his lap, holding me close and kissing me, providing excellent aftercare. We then headed to the guest room and continued to enjoy each other's bodies. He brought me to orgasm again and then I told him I wanted him.

As he entered me, it felt amazing and grew from there. It was incredible to feel so much pleasure the entire time he was inside me. Once we were both spent, we held each other, and the waves continued to undulate through my body. Ultimately, we decided to go to sleep, waking early enough to resume our sexploration before he had to go to work the next morning.

Sex is messy

Unlike what Hollywood would have us believe, sex is messy. Interestingly, as a counterpoint, I once read a novel in which the author deliberately wrote sex scenes that included periods, erectile dysfunction and other less-than-sexy/less-than-perfect encounters...aka real life. But, somehow even knowing that, it can be hard to let go of these pre-conceived notions of what sex should look like.

When we are with our primary or long-term partner, there is less of an issue and less awkwardness wondering if we're doing it "right," whatever that means. But, when you are with someone new that you don't know well, it can be hard to quiet the mind and not second guess if your actions (and reactions) are on point. Was I being too quiet? Too loud? Was I being clear that I liked (or disliked) what he was doing? Were my sounds a turn-on or turn-off?

And while we might have had a conversation about sexual preferences prior to climbing into bed with someone, you can't anticipate everything. Plus, although communication is key, you are not scripting a scene; you want to let go and be in the moment.

But that being said, I did think it would be prudent to find my voice in the moment and to communicate more clearly than I had been doing. To start asking: Do you like when I do this? Or would you prefer I do that? I really enjoy it when you touch me like [that], but less so when you do [that]. Sex certainly didn't need to be silent or without words; it just was not the time to have a discourse on western European politics or some other unrelated topic.

And, yes, sex does get messy. There are fluids; there are biological miscalculations; there is life which gets in the way (or not, if we welcome it). It becomes harder to plan out everything especially as your body is slowly changing. As a premenopausal woman, I bleed; I am she who bleeds but does not die! It is a powerful time, not a shameful one as I had been previously led to believe. No, I wasn't going to deliberately choose to be intimate with a new partner when I was at the height of my menstrual cycle. But things happen.

I had struggled with the concept of being messy for a long time, both inside and outside of the bedroom. During a boudoir photo shoot, I explored some of this discomfort with rose petals scattered everywhere, tousled hair and smudged make-up, all of which added to the allure and the freedom I felt in letting go and being in the moment.

After a passionate night of sex, I noticed blankets scattered on the floor, sheets in disarray, garments flung far and wide. We embrace the aftermath of those inanimate objects. Why not embrace the messiness of us humans too?

Perhaps it was much easier said than done. In this regard, we are often quick to blame ourselves, no matter what. Living in a world where the laws of the land coexist with the laws of nature, we seek justice when we feel such laws have been violated, wanting to inflict punishment to fit the crime, to rectify the wrongdoing. But we frequently misinterpret Newton's Third Law of Motion ("For every action, there is an equal and opposite reaction") and are often our own harshest judges.

Last Labor Day weekend, Viktor and I had spent a near perfect day at the beach. The weather was glorious, the water was divine, and we had a delicious dinner on our way back to the city. The next day we found ourselves back at work, intermittently slathering on aloe on our sunburnt skin. In addition to memories of our lovely day trip, we had the red, raw splotches marking our various body parts to show for it. Alas, a minor negative consequence of a happy occasion and we looked forward to our next beach excursion.

Meanwhile, a few months back, I had had a date with someone that had gone really well but had some weird consequences that struck me more intensely. We had had very pleasurable, penetrative sex a few times during our date, but on one of the occasions, he advised me that the condom had slipped off (he wasn't as erect as he needed to be) and gotten stuck inside me. I excused myself, went to the bathroom and felt around my vaginal canal, but didn't find or feel anything. Afterward he departed, I cleaned up and tossed out the used condoms and wrappers and forgot all about it...

Until two weeks later when I felt something slip out of me and into the toilet — it was the lost condom! OK, I was admittedly a bit freaked out, but apparently this is a thing that happens (at least according to the Internet). I checked in with the guy and we agreed that there was no cause for concern regarding STIs, so I planned to forget all about it...

Until I had a date with Dash (who happens to be a medical doctor) who suggested, on the morning after our sexual encounter, that I might have BV[7]. Not romantic, but I suppose I shouldn't complain about free medical advice and a doctor that makes house calls.

Although BV isn't a serious condition and can occur as a consequence of things unrelated to sexual intercourse, mine was likely caused as a result of the condom being stuck in my vaginal canal for such a lengthy period of time. Still, I felt gross and, much like Hester Prynne's scarlet letter A, I felt branded with the initials BV. I berated myself for having let this happen — as if it were entirely my fault. Moreover, I felt like I had committed a "crime" and was being punished for my "sins." The "sin" of being a sexual being!

---

[7] BV or Bacterial vaginosis is defined by The Mayo Clinic as: "[A] type of vaginal inflammation caused by the overgrowth of bacteria naturally found in the vagina, which upsets the natural balance."

The next day, I went to my primary care provider to confirm the diagnosis, researched my treatment options, talked about it with a few girlfriends and then, thankfully, moved on.

But it was telling that I was so swift to blame myself and felt universally judged (or more correctly, judged by the universe) for my sexual actions while I felt no remorse at not having applied sunscreen as sufficiently as I should have at the beach. Life is all about action and reaction — our actions have consequences. But, in reality, such consequences were not judgements; they were simply consequences.

As women, we are often quick to find fault and judge ourselves when it came to our sexual activities even if we were enjoying ourselves at the time and felt comfortable in the moment. We paint ourselves with the broad brushes of shame, disgust, regret, doubt and, dare I say it...slut.

Yet, there was no crime committed. The condom incident and resulting BV were unfortunate, short-lived consequences of a sexual encounter between two consenting adults. Neither the universe nor any other force was punishing me. I just had to learn to stop punishing myself.

And yet, I continued to do so...

Polyamorous, it's right there in the title: poly = many. But how many was too many?

Before I got married, I had had 10 sexual partners including Viktor. Some of those were one-night stands, but most were in the context of a dating relationship. And that was over a period of seven years. So, once I was a married monogamous woman, I figured that my number would never change, nor did it matter.

But obviously things had changed. When we first opened up our marriage, sex (specifically intercourse) seemed so scary and I considered it to be a Very Big Deal. Thus, my play was limited to outercourse. Then, a few months in, with Viktor's blessing, I chose to have sex with Jake during our first full swap.

Since then, I had had penetrative sex with several other partners, with the expectation that there was some sort of ongoing relationship with the person. In some cases, that didn't turn out as expected, but one can't plan for everything.

Now that the number of partners was growing, I was feeling uncomfortable about the number. Like really uncomfortable. And, I had been trying to figure out why I was feeling so uncomfortable. Why should I care about a number? Do other polyamorous people think about such things? Part of the general nature of open relationships is that the number of partners will not stay constant.

I questioned myself, wondering if I was being too permissive with my body and had a lot of "shoulds" swirling through my head. I should be more... (discriminate?) I should be less... (of a slut?) As I continued to think about it, I realized that while there was some validity to my concerns, more truthfully, this was simply shame rearing its ugly head again!

The question was: How did I reconcile a sexual lifestyle that focused on the many with my desire to not feel such shame around my choices? There was no black and white answer to this question. Rather, I needed to be clear with myself as to what I wanted in both the short term and long term.

So, what did I want? I wanted connection; I wanted stimulating conversations; I wanted ongoing relationships. I didn't want to sleep around for the sake of sleeping around. I didn't want to feel used. I had started to put together a list of qualifiers, but I really didn't think that made sense either; to set parameters such as having at least one real date was arbitrary and not really the point.

So where did I go from here? First of all, I stopped counting. Numbers didn't matter; they just messed with my head! Rather, intention mattered. Authenticity mattered. Desire mattered. The only thing I wanted less of was shame; that was the only thing that counted!

I regret nothing

Life is equally messy as I soon learned. In this regard, my fifth erotic party was yet again another adventure filled with unexpected plot twists and turns. On one of our dates, after I had shared my experiences at previous play parties, Patrick expressed an interest in attending and had asked me if I would like to go with him as a couple. I immediately replied yes and looked forward to the event. This time the theme was Alice in Wonderland: Down the Bunny Hole. I asked him: "Alice or Queen of Hearts?" Patrick replied: "Alice," to which Viktor then told me that he no longer liked Patrick — but he was only kidding.

The Best Laid Plans of Mice and Men...

Despite that dialogue, in the lead up to the event, I actually decided that the Queen of Hearts was more my style and had fun planning my costume. A few days before the party, Patrick and I met for coffee to discuss our intentions and desires for the event. We agreed that full nudity and intercourse at the party were not on the menu because I hadn't felt comfortable with this idea at the other parties. The thought of being so vulnerable in such a public space filled with me dread, not desire. We also determined that we were going to go together but with the understanding that we would be free to hang out separately on occasion and that we would check in with one another as the evening proceeded.

I also told Patrick about Ryan. He had heard about my Shibari suspension session with Ryan at the February party, but I now impressed upon him that things had progressed further, and he seemed okay with it, picking up on the way I talked about Ryan. I also advised Patrick that Jake and Mia would be at the party so he wouldn't be blindsided, as I had had a text from them earlier in the evening, letting me know that they would be in attendance.

The day of the party Patrick came to my apartment as planned. He looked great in his Mad Hatter-themed attire. We ordered sushi and I had gotten us a bottle of sake to enjoy with our meal as we kicked off the night in a festive mood. After dinner, we got a car service to take us to the party.

Upon arrival in Brooklyn, I introduced Patrick to the party hosts and, soon after, he met Ryan, Jake and Mia. It was both exhilarating and weird to be commingled with these people in one room but, not surprisingly, I liked the attention. Plus, I was very eager to see Ryan after having had such an amazing time with him earlier in the week with our Shibari scene.

As we had agreed, Patrick and I spent the early part of the party interacting with a few people, enjoying the wine I had brought, hanging out by the fire pit and then partaking of the ritual together. After the ritual, Ryan was available and proceeded to tie and suspend me while Patrick looked on. I felt torn between immersing myself in the experience with Ryan and ensuring that I gave Patrick sufficient attention. I occasionally made eye contact with Patrick in an attempt to balance the two competing thoughts.

Once Ryan had untied the ropes and released me, I headed back over to Patrick and we began to kiss and then touch each other more explicitly. I focused on what I was feeling in the moment and was having fun, but when I started to hear myself moaning softly, I became very self-conscious and asked him to stop, which he did. We went back outside to the fire pit and held each other, intermittently talking and kissing.

At some point, Ryan came over and privately asked if I was okay. I told him I was, but that I would rather be with him than Patrick. He said he would contrive for all three of us to be together and I readily agreed to this plan.

So, I finally did it. I had sex...at a sex party! Not long after, we were all back downstairs, with Ryan leading me, Mia and Patrick to the mattresses. We all started kissing and fondling one another. Mia was kissing me, Patrick was touching my breasts, Ryan was holding my hand and I was stroking Mia's breasts. It was fantastic. Then Mia left and I had the attention of the two men, shifting periodically to kiss one and then the other, while taking turns reaching for their cocks.

A while later, Ryan pulled off my panties and went down on me. Around this time, Patrick departed the threesome, leaving me and Ryan alone together. I let him go and turned my full attention to Ryan. The world slipped away just like when we were in the pool. I wasn't aware of the crowds or the noise or anything else. There was only Ryan and me in that moment and then we were having sex. I didn't feel self-conscious or uncomfortable. Perhaps some of it was due to me not being completely nude — I was still wearing my bra, harness/garters and stockings. I only knew that I really wanted him and didn't want to stop despite my previous trepidation.

Eventually Ryan and I took a break and we agreed I would go find Patrick. Once I found him, I asked him if he minded that I wanted to spend more time with Ryan. He asked if I wanted to go home with Ryan and at that moment, I really didn't know what I wanted and told him that I just wanted to spend more time with Ryan for now.

Patrick said he would leave. I felt badly and knew that this wasn't what either of us had had in mind when we planned and discussed our intentions, but I couldn't deny what I was feeling, I couldn't fake or manufacture desire for Patrick that I wasn't feeling nor would I make myself do something I didn't want to do even if it felt like something a good girl should do. I had done enough of that in the past — sacrificing myself for someone else's ego, desire, etc. I loved myself and my body too much now to do that ever again.

So, while there was a pang of guilt and regret for potentially hurting Patrick — which was not my intention — I pushed past it and let it go.

I knew that I cared about him, but also knew that I didn't have an obligation to anyone but myself. I was honest and transparent and while I might have been able to handle the situation slightly differently, I didn't know that it would have been better; just different.

While waiting for Ryan to return, I was hanging out with Jake and Mia and then Jake was telling Mia that he wanted to be with me. I wasn't exactly sure what he meant but then suddenly he was pulling me toward the mattress area, and I found myself obediently following him. We started to play, and he went down on me, but I realized that I wasn't really into it. Yes, I had enjoyed being with Jake in the past but in that instance, I really just wasn't feeling it. Jake said I look tired and I admitted that I didn't really want to be having sex with him. I apologized and he teased me a bit for apologizing but mostly because he cared about me not because of my decision.

I kissed Jake goodbye and returned to Ryan. We eventually resumed our intimacy and play and had sex, which was, once again, incredibly orgasmic for me. We spent the remainder of the night entwined in one another at the fire pit before we decided to call it a night.

I grabbed a Lyft home and was eventually joined at home by Viktor, who had been at a rave all night. We quickly updated each other on our respective evenings and then found a final burst of energy to enjoy each other before drifting off to sleep.

But, in reflecting on my night, I realized that I had gone along to go along for so long. Why? Because it was easier and less fraught with conflict, but in the end it was destructive. I was finally getting better at listening to my body and telling my head to shut up. I was feeling into what I really wanted and not simply doing what was expected of me as a friend, a wife, a date or a lover. And it felt really good.

I still didn't have a good reason for why I felt so uninterested in Patrick on Saturday night. He hadn't done anything wrong. I just felt less desire or lust in that direction. Was it exclusively due to Ryan's presence? I didn't know. I did reach out to Patrick to apologize for any hurt I may have caused and for the night turning out differently than we had anticipated. I wasn't sure if he wanted to see me again, but I left it up to him. I really liked him and thought he was an awesome person. But perhaps I had put him in the "friend zone" as a result of so many dinner dates and fewer opportunities to be intimate. I truly wasn't sure.

Regardless, I was less concerned about my confusion and was more concerned about feeling into and honoring my desire. This was new territory for me, and I was embracing what I felt as I navigated various situations and experiences.

Over time, I had been busy meeting people and dating. There had been a lot of movement and, consequently, numerous learning experiences. But where did I hope to go? Now that it had been several months since I had met Jon, Patrick and Ryan (among others), I started to wonder about what to expect as things moved forward. These relationships had preceded so differently than my initial venture into dating.

Whereas I had seen Hank a handful of times over a three-month period that first summer, I had now seen John and Patrick five times each in as many weeks (and had seen Ryan three times in a week and a half). Things were moving more quickly and more intensely, but it felt more real and authentic as our time had given us the opportunity to get to know one another, not just simply have sex. I really liked the idea of growing these relationships further — building upon our initial intimacy, understanding each other's bodies and exploring kinks, desires and turn-ons.

And, likely because I was a planner with regard to all things, I wondered at which point did these relationships become established. Was there an unwritten compact to simply keep meeting up until you decided not to?

But I did think about the consequences of such attachments. No, I didn't love these men nor was I in love with any of them, but at first, I had no attachment to the outcome of our dates. Now, I felt a connection and enjoyed having each of them *specifically* in my life. And

I felt that I was more apt to second guess myself with my text messages now that I feared the potential loss if I said or wrote the "wrong" thing. How much should I say and reveal about what I was thinking and feeling? I opted for the truth.

Further, I questioned if there was a danger in getting too close; in caring too much? If so, where was that line? I didn't know. These entanglements were so different from the types of relationships I had had when I was dating before marriage because, of course, the "end game" was so different. In general, I knew I had the tendency to overthink or overanalyze. I knew that I needed to simply enjoy the ride and take each date for what it brought and not worry about tomorrow or next week.

I suppose this was where the swingers' lifestyle was "cleaner" than the poly lifestyle in that those encounters were more usually one-offs, not cumulative dating experiences. And yet, I wanted to get to know these partners better, to explore and be truly seen, not to rotate through a string of strangers.

Regardless, my constant was and always would be Viktor. I admitted that I had gotten caught up in the excitement of all of these men. It felt good to be wanted. But, if I allowed myself to get too distracted by having new guys, I ran the risk of not paying sufficient and meaningful attention to Viktor; that was not what I wanted. I did crave the ardor and attention of these other men; the attention fed me. It fueled my turn-on and desire. I could exist without it and them but, for now, I didn't want to.

Overall, it felt good to learn about myself in this way and to have found myself on this long, overdue journey. I was really excited with the way that things had unfolded and looked forward to seeing what came next, whether with Jon, Patrick, Ryan or with others. Most importantly, I had stepped out of my comfort zone and stepped into my sexuality — truly owning it unapologetically and that, was everything!

These revelations reverberated throughout my life, not just my dating life. The next week, in my S Factor class, my teacher called me a Super Goddess and talked about how I had been revealing and, standing for, my truth over these past few months in class. It was perfectly timed feedback since she had also shared with us about the arrival of the New Moon that night and our ability to set intentions for our future desires.

Interestingly, when I got out of class, there was an email from Viktor, who had coincidentally forwarded me an article about the New Moon. As I read the article, I was profoundly struck by this statement:

"At the same time, we may be questioning what outmoded commitments and obligations are holding us back that we now need to break. However, this period is not about running away. Aries the Ram is confrontational, and we're learning to face each other — to confront our feelings so we can work through the messier, illogical aspects of our lives and relationships."
— *Alchemist's Kitchen*

In addition to the New Moon synchronicity, this discussion was also apropos because I had reached out to Patrick the night before. After everything that had happened (or perhaps hadn't happened) with Patrick at the last erotic party, I didn't know precisely where things stood with him. I had followed up with him immediately after the event to apologize and received a brief response. Then, just prior to heading out on vacation, I asked him if I was persona non grata; he noted that he was not like that and wished me the best on our trip. However, I still didn't know if he wanted to resume our relationship or not. And, frankly, I wasn't sure what I wanted from him either. I just knew that things felt unfinished and I wanted to know his thoughts at the very least.

So, I sent him a text, indicating that I didn't know what he wanted and was thus leaving it to him to reach out if and when he was interested. He wrote back the next morning:

"Good morning! It's been a pleasure to get to know you, and I hope to see you around the neighborhood. But I'm not interested in being intimate again. Here's why: In our conversations ahead of the party you set several clear boundaries, and I'm happy to have held those. But then I watched you enthusiastically blow past all of them. Which was your choice, of course. But that choice included a break of trust — for me at least, and maybe for others. And that's a big turn-off."

I shared his text with Viktor who immediately asked me how I felt about Patrick's response. Admittedly, there was a brief sting (no one ever wants to be considered a turn-off), but I definitely understood and appreciated his perspective and feelings and certainly respected his honesty. Moreover, I felt that it was a fair assessment of what had actually happened.

I further acknowledged to Viktor that his response made it easier to figure out how to go forward because I wasn't sure I was sufficiently attracted to him if he had wanted to continue, even though I really liked him as a person. In looking back, I realized that I was feeling less of a pull to him even in the car on the way to the party, which should have been a red flag, but there was nothing I could have done at that point anyway, even if I had been aware of it.

And Patrick was spot on that it had been a break of trust even though he didn't know the true extent of it. Yes, there had been a break of trust between Patrick and me, but there had also been one between Viktor and me. Before the event, I had initially agreed not to have sex at a play party without Viktor, but while I consented to this stipulation, it was really only because I didn't have any desire to have sex with Patrick at the party, not that I necessarily believed in this rule.

In reality, I knew that Viktor's prohibition was an ego thing; he didn't want me to give something to someone that I hadn't already given to him, but I didn't take the time to unpack that with him at the time, thinking we could address it at another, more relevant, time.

But, at the party, in the heat of the moment, I chose what I wanted to do based on what felt right to me and my body and not to anyone else. I felt into my desire and surrendered to it, all the while knowing that it was a breach of trust. And, although I believed that the fact that it was someone Viktor knew (and really liked) would mitigate, but not absolve, the situation, I recognized that I had broken my promise.

So, as soon as I arrived home, I confessed what had happened. Yes, understandably, and justifiably, Viktor was upset, but he listened and heard me and saw the truth and honesty of my apology as well. We agreed to continue to revisit and talk about the situation, but we were able to move on in a loving way.

In the wake of all of that, Viktor felt that Patrick's response was interesting because Viktor had come around to my decision to follow my own desire, yet also saw Patrick's point regarding the trust issue. Viktor and I continued to text back and forth about the topic, further united in how we viewed the encounter and even more connected to one another.

As the day progressed, I thought more and more about Patrick's message. I also took time to reflect on what had happened at the party and realized with stark clarity that I never had had any shame or regret at the conclusion of the party. The most interesting thing about what had happened at the party was that I never regretted my actions!

Yes, I had felt very badly about hurting Patrick and recognized that my behavior toward him had not been as upstanding as I would have liked (although I realized that the context of bringing a date to a sex party was vastly different than bringing a date to dinner or the theater, so I was not going to beat myself up about it). But the revelation that I didn't feel badly about what I had *chosen* to do was so freeing! Wow!

Further, I recognized the duality between following my desires, especially at a sex party, versus holding firm to (somewhat arbitrary?) boundaries. Could you really script desire?

Yes, I had set boundaries for myself before heading to the party, but things could change in the moment. Over the past several years, I had been pushing my boundaries (particularly in, and as a result of, my classes with Mama Gena), so it stood to reason that I was going to push them as I continued to explore my sexuality, especially in the context of a sex party. Equally notable was that I followed my body instead of my head for a change!

Finally, while I acknowledged that a break of trust with anyone was not a great idea and noted that my actions may have been inadvertently hurtful, the flip side was that no one had really ever cared about the fallout when I had broken trust with myself — such as by having sex when I didn't want to. Rather, I was so thrilled that for once I had maintained trust with the most important person: ME! For a change, I was true to me!

So, as I reflected on all that had happened as a result of this one night, I was more committed than ever to standing for MY TRUTH. I was so delighted to be on this journey to better understand my desire and to be open to exploring what felt right in the moment. I trusted myself, fully, for the first time!

Lessons learned

For various reasons, I had been feeling a bit off for about a week or so. In fact, there was almost an anxious, manic feeling and I felt driven to do something, but wasn't sure what to do.

Among the things I did, was to return to the dating app in the hope of finding a date for the weekend since Viktor would be at raves on both Friday and Saturday nights. I was eager to explore D/s in a more formal way, so finding a Dom was of particular interest.

After some chatting, I made plans to meet up with a number of men, but two of the three dates were cancelled. And, I had a weird virtual Dom from Ireland/possible scam incident, which was unsettling. I was emotionally charged but was trying to push through as if everything was fine.

In this somewhat altered state, I attended an event with Kasia Urbaniak of The Academy: Fearless Desires. Among her pearls of wisdom, she noted that you felt real, true embodied desire in the body as sensation, emotion, mood and that it doesn't go away; it takes our attention until it is met, and you have no say in what you want. Her message really struck home with me and I felt even more vulnerable and fragile. Later on, I came across a Faccbook post highlighting the need to put attention and energy on what you wished to manifest. Okay, Universe, message received loud and clear!

On Saturday morning, Viktor and I finally took the time to connect and I was able to share with him all that had been coming up for me, the tumble and jumble of emotions, questions, concerns, unmet desires and fears. I cried for a bit and felt calmer and more settled as he held me close.

Then, Viktor asked if I wanted to watch some Erica Lust or get tied up by him. I chose the latter and we soon headed to the bedroom, where he proceeded to secure me to the bedposts, gave me a sensual massage and then fucked me intensely. It was insanely hot, erotic and pleasurable! Afterward, I felt so much better! Little did I know what our sexcapade had unleashed.

In my post-sex glow, I primped and pampered myself as I got ready for my date. We had a really nice time getting to know each other and agreed to go out again. The positive experience really fed and filled me, fueling my further preparations as I headed home to metamorphose into a bunny in time for the erotic party's Playboy Mansion theme.

On my way to the party, there was a flurry of messages from Jon and some of the dating app flakes (aka those who had started and stopped conversations from a week-plus ago). I realized that something had shifted in my energy.

When I arrived at the party, I immediately connected with Jake and Mia, with whom I had been texting earlier in the week. Jake had been encouraging me to attend, which I had decided to do at the last minute, when I was asked to perform a sensual dance at the event. I was pleasantly surprised to see Ryan at the party, as I didn't think he would be there.

While chatting with Mia, she introduced me to Dash. Dash and his wife, Dahlia, were relatively new to the lifestyle and were very intrigued with Viktor's and my story. I was eager to talk with them about their experiences and desires and to share mine with them. Plus, Dahlia was incredibly sexy and beautiful! And Dash mentioned that she was into women.

Then, it was time for the ritual and my dance. It was always intoxicating for me to dance; to feel the attention and gaze of the audience, but also to feel the way my body moved and connected with the music.

After my performance, Ryan asked me if he could replace my bodysuit with a rope "corset" and have me walk around as an "advertisement" for his Shibari skills. I initially joked that I needed to take a second edible to do so, but then readily agreed, removed my leotard and proceeded to let him tie me up. He threaded the rope around my neck, crisscrossed it in diamond pattern down my body, sliding it between my legs. I felt the constriction of the rope as it pulled on my torso; it was slightly uncomfortable, yet very erotic. I dutifully went off to showcase Ryan's work, surprised at how comfortable I felt to be so nude and vulnerable in just rope and a thong.

After spending time with Tim, whom I hadn't seen in several months, I reconnected with Dash and Dahlia. As the three of us talked, Dash suggested that we continue our conversation horizontally, so we went back downstairs and found a comfortable place on the mattresses. We shared and talked openly, and then we began to kiss and caress each other. Still bound, my range of motion was somewhat stifled, and I felt a bit like I was wearing a chastity belt.

At some point, Ryan came to check on me and released me from my literal bondage. I continued to explore Dash and Dahlia's bodies, enjoying the touch and feel of them both and enjoyed receiving their touches as well now that my body was freed from its restraints. Eventually I took a break from them and wandered off, running into Jake who made good on his promise to give me a very pleasurable, erotic massage.

A little while later, Dash and Dahlia were getting ready to leave and offered me a ride home, which I gratefully accepted (having desired to conjure a ride home before I even got to the party).

I arrived home in a state of bliss, further enhanced by seeing a slew of texts from various admirers. I then responded to an earlier text from Viktor who was on his way home from a rave, so I stayed up so I could share my night with him. We fell into bed exhausted after such an amazing day, clearly having made magic once again!

With magic still in the air, I had a profound dance at S Factor during an Erotic Creature Romp, a four-hour, immersive workshop. During my first dance, I had my hands tied behind my back. It felt thrilling as I strained against the binds, yearning to touch, to break free... and the vulnerability of being bound and restrained. I pulled against the taut strings; it was like music being drawn out slowly through the air. I felt the raw depth of forcing my body into new shapes, breaking old and stagnant patterns and pushing against bonds and boundaries.

Then, in my next dance, I changed my outfit and style of music and preceded to explore the Dangerous Challenger Erotic Creature icon whose core emotion was anger. But, as my teacher explained, it was not just anger for the sake of anger, but anger that needed to be met.

I donned my patent leather, thigh-high boots; a ripped, red top; a sexy black skirt; and kept on my stretchy, elastic harness. I climbed the pole and waited for the music to start, unsure what to expect. As Karmin's voice pierced the silence, I became electric. The shock and awe of wielding a chain, first as a belt and then as a weapon as it loudly clanged on the floor, fueled my energy, my heat, my turn-on and my power!

Afterwards, my teacher reflected back my dance to me seeing a parallel between the two. This latter dance was a continuation of the first, she said. You wanted to provoke, asking the observer: What are you going to do about it? The "it" being both my rage and my passion. And what did I want? She suggested that I wanted to be tied up. I didn't doubt her assessment.

My exploration into Shibari, first with Viktor, my equally erotic encounters with Ryan, and also the use of restraints with Jake and Mia, had been intense and beautiful, allowing me to expand in so many ways as I surrendered and sought attention to truly be seen.

Being seen. I kept coming back to this. I wanted people to really see me. But to what purpose? As the lyrics from Red's "The Ever" stated,

"But you saw more
You saw my deepest part
With the light of a thousand stars
You saw them awake in me"

Sexually, I thought it harkened back to how I wanted to be fucked. If you really saw me (and got me), you would presumably know the answer without having to ask.

There was a real truth here that required and deserved more exploration, reflection and experience. I felt that I had tapped into something very telling. And the dance sparked a new fantasy: the Dom who becomes the sub. How hot was that?

With my interest in D/s growing, I was eager to engage in more encounters of power exchange. I had met Brady back in April and we had a fun, first date. We had bonded over cocktails, which led to an intense (and inappropriate) make-out session at an uptown lounge. When he expressed his desire to go out again, he indicated that he would prefer to go somewhere with more privacy (so as not to shock fellow patrons again) and shared that he wanted to spend more time with my sexy persona. I readily agreed and we picked a date for the following month given our mutually busy schedules.

We had arranged to meet at an upscale bar, which gave us the opportunity to reconnect after the four-week hiatus. I had been more casually dressed for our first date, so I made up for my error with an overtly sexy, black and nude-colored, lace cocktail dress, which very much met with Brady's approval.

Over drinks, Brady brought up the topic of a safe word and stated that it would be... safeword. I knew from our first date that he was into spanking, but we hadn't discussed much else in the way of D/s play, so I wasn't sure what to expect. Plus, this was only our second time meeting each other, so I was both excited and nervous at the same time about what was in store.

We finished our drinks and headed over to the Roosevelt Hotel lobby bar where Brady ordered us a second round. As we sipped our cocktails, Brady handed me a room key and told me there was something on the bed that he wanted me to have. I headed upstairs, opened the door and was greeted with a note and a leather collar. I gingerly fingered the leather on the collar and then reached for, and read, the note.

"There's only one decision you have to make this evening: to put on this collar or not. If you do, it means you belong to me tonight. You're my courtesan, and the only thing you have to worry about is my pleasure. You will do as you're told, and if you make me happy you will be rewarded. If you don't, you'll be punished. It all depends on what I decide. If that's what you want, have the courage to put this on and come back to me in the bar."

It was a very titillating invitation. I put away the note, took a deep breath and fastened the collar around my neck. Then I grabbed the key, shut the door and returned to the bar. I didn't know if anyone else noticed my new "necklace" but Brady was pleased to see me wearing it.

We finished up in the bar and went back up to the room together. I was to call him "Sir" and he would address me as his "little pet." His first request was for me to take off my dress. I unzipped it and let it fall to the floor. I was then asked to sit on his lap, which I dutifully obeyed. Next, he wanted me to place my face against his hard cock so I could see how my obedience turned him on. Eventually I was asked to remove his clothing and then kiss, not lick or suck, his penis.

We then walked over to the bed to continue our mutual seduction. The outercourse was intense and orgasmic as he repeatedly tasted me, teased my nipples and otherwise brought me to climax. After several hours of play, we fell asleep, waking up with the first rays of sunlight. In the early morning hours, we resumed our exploration of one another.

Admittedly, I wasn't sure if the scene continued from one day to the next, so I continued to request permission and referred to him as Sir. Interestingly, there had been no impact play. Perhaps I had been too obedient and hadn't warranted a spanking? I wasn't sure but hoped for a debrief at some point.

By 7:30 a.m., I was dressed and ready to head home to walk the dog. Before I left, Brady unfastened the collar and then presented it to me, saying that he wanted me to keep it and that it should serve as a reminder whether I had it on (or not) that I belonged to him during future encounters.

He accompanied me downstairs and outside as we said goodbye and I returned to real life.

But, while Elvis crooned, "A little less conversation, a little more action, please" and also — funnily enough in this context — went on to ask for "more bite" and "less fight," it was not exactly a recipe for success in BDSM (Bondage/Domination-submission/Sadism/Masochism).

Admittedly, although Viktor and I had taken a full-day course with professional Dominant, Om Rupani, once upon a time, we were still relatively new to the scene. And I was more aware of my naivete as I reflected on my encounter with Brady.

As I traveled home from our date, Brady texted me to thank me for a lovely evening and added, "Next time. Hopefully soon." Nearly two weeks passed without comment, so I sent him a quick "Happy Friday." He responded later that day, at which point I advised him that I was surprised not to have heard from him for a debrief of our scene. He apologized for the lack of communication, citing an upcoming work deadline along with planned travel.

While I acknowledged and respected his busy schedule, I pushed back on my request for a debrief. He agreed and promised to be in touch after his trip and followed up accordingly. We arranged to meet for a drink on a Saturday afternoon at the King Cole Bar (he apparently had a love of classic New York City hotels).

Soon after we arrived, we dove into the conversation. He immediately revealed that he wasn't interested in pursuing anything further with me but was open to discussing the scene. He further admitted that he was really surprised by my request and my reference to it as a "debrief." It was clear that although he fancied himself a Dom, he really wasn't that experienced or knowledgeable about proper practices.

However, as we continued to talk, the importance of such aftercare really hit home for him. I explained that I had been uncomfortable because I hadn't known when the scene was supposed to end and that we hadn't really discussed our mutual desires and expectations. We had never set any ground rules or boundaries. Moreover, while I had known that he liked spanking from his dating app profile, that hadn't been a part of our activities and I really hadn't known what he had or hadn't wanted from me over the course of the night.

Once he recognized how his actions (or rather the lack thereof) had impacted our scene and safety, Brady apologized profusely and owned his mistakes. And I took responsibility for my part as well. Overall, we agreed that his desire to get to know me so quickly after only one date was too much, too soon. And, that an in-depth negotiation should have taken place well before I put on that collar. So, we completed our conversation, bid each other goodbye and went our separate ways. But you bet I kept the collar!

While I was a little disappointed to say goodbye to Brady, I was more disappointed to give up the idea of a D/s relationship. I had clearly been seeking such an arrangement for some time as evidenced by other potential connections and matches on the app that had, as yet yielded nothing, along with my initial, positive responses to being tied up and surrendering to another's power.

However, I soon matched with Gary who had significant experience and knowledge in the D/s scene. In fact, while I was unaware of this until we met face-to-face, he actually taught classes around the city and planned to write an instructional guidebook on the subject.

Needless to say, he was aghast when I shared my Brady story with him, but thankfully he recognized that I was aware of my mistakes and would be much wiser going forward. We had a lovely first date at a wine bar near Union Square and talked through our interests and desires in connection with life in general and BDSM in particular.

Fittingly, I had had a conversation with Tova earlier in the day which had helped me reflect on my previous D/s experiences and get clarity on my desires for such interactions in the future. I had shared with her an interesting point I had read that afternoon, which talked about BDSM practitioners requiring more intellectual (as opposed to animal) stimulation with regard to their sexual arousal.

I also realized that the past D/s scenes with Viktor had only scratched the surface due to our lack of experience and knowledge, but also perhaps due to the equal nature of our day-to-day relationship. Given that Gary was both new to me and well versed in these arts, I was eager to explore this side of myself in a safe, sane, consensual way. As someone who had significant difficulty relaxing and letting go (in all things), I was especially intrigued about the concept of subspace —

entering into an altered psychological state as a result of the experience.[8]

After our first date, Gary and I were both eager for me to explore BDSM together. Due to travel and other commitments, it was three weeks before we next met, but in the interim, there was a lot of texting back and forth. Some of it was simply planning logistics, but Gary gave me lots of information in the lead up to our date. He sent me images of various implements that he had at his disposal such as canes and paddles. However, he talked a lot about floggers and implied that this particular tool might be the key for me to really get into subspace.

His communication increased in frequency and intensity as the day got closer. In fact, on the actual day of our date, the texts came more often and became more explicit, building excitement and anticipation. Starting at noon (we were meeting at 6:00 p.m.), he began to count down the hours, sending a text on the hour, every hour, and connecting the number of hours with something sexual. With two hours to go, there was an extremely visceral response within my body to his text, "2.... words Yes Sir" at 5:00 p.m. I was already looking forward to the date but now, I was even more excited (and turned on!) to see him.

We first met up at my local wine bar for a nice meal before heading to my apartment. At dinner and then afterward, we continued to tease out the details of what was to come. We had agreed to a medley of activities that started with an "Intro to Impact Play 101." Knowing that this was a new and deliberate exploration, Gary took an intentionally academic approach and explained each implement from straps and paddles to hairbrushes, floggers and canes. Then we selected an assortment of tools for him to use on me. I disrobed and revealed my *ouvert* panty, which he was pleased to see, as he applied each one to my bare bottom.

---

[8] For a good description of this altered state, please see:
http://thejourneyofwill.blogspot.com/2012/12/two-kinds-of-subspace.html

Gary had given me green, yellow and red to use as my safe words, but, at times when I was quieter, he assured me that he could read my body/body language loud and clear. For the most part, I enjoyed the sensations, but, on occasion, the pain was a bit sharp, veering on the red side of yellow.

After the initial impact demonstration was over, we shifted to other activities involving dominance. Gary applied nipple and labia clamps, used a vibrator on my clit and applied additional slaps to my ass. By now I was very aroused and very much enjoying the experience. Finally, after ascertaining that impact play was not my true kink (Gary noted that it pulled me out of my body and into my head), he said I would be a fun submissive. I replied that I hoped he found me fun now!

We then turned our attention to each other. We talked about orgasms and Gary admitted that he couldn't wait to fuck me and added that he had been wanting to ever since he first saw me. I was quite eager to be with him by then and his words pushed me further. As we proceeded to have sex, it was incredibly orgasmic from the initial moment of penetration and we played with several different positions, which were both fun and informative.

Both fully sated, Gary spent a lot of time holding me afterwards, providing and modeling good after care. Before leaving, he expressed desire to see me again for further exploration and I readily consented. Since he had a wife and girlfriend, I told him I was happy to remain in his orbit as a satellite, but Gary assured me that I was most definitely a planet!

It was an incredible experience, and I was grateful to have made this connection as I continued to truly explore my BDSM interests. I was now even more convinced that this was the gateway to my true surrender.

In the days that followed, Gary and I continued to text back and forth. He asked me to forgive him for still being caught up in our encounter, but there was no need for forgiveness as I felt it too. There was a lingering connectedness between us. It was so different from falling in love or even in lust; it felt new and unique, but very enjoyable.

A few days after our engagement, we had spoken about sending each other energy, so while I self-pleasured one night, I distinctly thought of him. The result was that I woke him from a dream! And even though I couldn't explain it adequately, I was delighted by this connection and very much looked forward to our continued exploration.

It's a matter of trust

Other explorations added to my knowledge as I learned additional lessons and vocabulary. Like the rest of the world, the dating scene was filled with acronyms. I frequently found myself heading over to the Urban Dictionary to decode people's profiles. It was a good thing I did because on one occasion I thought that a duo who described themselves as a "VGL couple" might be vegan lovers, but it turned out that VGL stood for <u>V</u>ery <u>G</u>ood <u>L</u>ooking (although if you have to state that you are very good looking...).

Another important acronym I learned was ENM: <u>E</u>thical <u>N</u>on-<u>M</u>onogamy. These three letters told an important story because it was essentially the difference between being truthful with your partner or being a cheater (yes, this was an oversimplification, but you get the idea).

On the dating apps, Viktor and I had connected profiles, so it was clear to potential partners that we were practicing ethical non-monogamy. Moreover, when I had met people at play parties or elsewhere, I was quick to let them know that I was married and was happy to explain our situation. I didn't want anyone to be accidentally misled or be surprised. If they were not interested in pursuing me further as a result, no worries, but I wanted to be upfront and honest from the start.

Moreover, from the very beginning of this journey, Viktor and I had shared everything. I told him every minute detail and, even when there were times that I was afraid to tell him what had happened, I spoke the truth. So, I was thrown by what happened with Dash and Dahlia when we next met up.

I had met Dash and Dahlia at one of the play parties earlier in the year, having been introduced to them by a mutual friend who confirmed my married, yet open, status. Similarly, since I met them together at an erotic event, it was obvious that they were married and, in the lifestyle, although they admitted to being very new to it. We all had a great time playing together at the party and I then enjoyed meeting up with Dash again a few weeks later. Dash and I had met for drinks, gone dancing and then came back to my apartment where we had sex and he spent the night.

After my date with Dash, I didn't hear from him for a few weeks, so I sent a simple hello. He responded relatively quickly, and we traded a few texts. Eventually he expressed interest in getting together again and offered up a date for him, Dahlia and me to connect.

Our plan was for me to meet them at their hotel (they were staying in New York City overnight), head somewhere for a nice dinner and/or drinks and then I was invited to join them in their room. Dash emphasized that the evening was to be about both of us; in his words, "two very beautiful, fun women." I was very much looking forward to our evening and was especially eager to see Dahlia again.

About two hours before we were supposed to meet up, Dash texted to confirm our timing and then dropped a bit of a bombshell. He confessed that he had never shared our sexual liaison with Dahlia! What? Not cool, dude!

I seriously contemplated cancelling, but 1) I was extremely excited about seeing Dahlia again and 2) I'm human. I simply expressed my displeasure at the situation and promised him my silence. Throughout the evening, I felt uncomfortable and had to watch what I said so as not to reveal Dash's secret.

After dinner and then drinks at the hotel's rooftop bar, we headed to their room. I mostly focused my attention on Dahlia and enjoyed kissing her and then slowly undressing her. Things proceeded well enough. I was having a pleasurable time with the two of them, however, when it was clear that I was about to go down on Dahlia, Dash immediately stopped me, saying, "She's not ready for that."

I admit that I should have been more explicit in asking for her enthusiastic consent before I ventured downward, but I felt very weird at being stopped not by Dahlia, but by Dash. Why couldn't she tell me what she did or didn't want herself? Then, a little later, while listening to the music that Dahlia had put on earlier, a song came on that apparently had meaning for them and Dahlia requested silence from all of us as it played.

So, three strikes (lies, creepy control and misty music) and I was out of there. I got dressed, politely said goodbye and headed home. They texted me the next day expressing their pleasure at having had their first threesome, which I appreciated, but I was resolved not to see them again. I just couldn't continue to perpetuate the lie, nor was I comfortable with their dynamic.

Meanwhile, as a counterpoint to this, I had recently started seeing Matt, whom I met on a dating app. I was drawn to his profile because he clearly stated his desire for ongoing contact and just genuinely seemed to be a really nice guy.

After some sweet text exchanges, we met in person at a speakeasy in the Gramercy Park area for light bites and drinks. We connected and enjoyed open, honest conversations right from the beginning. We then left the speakeasy and walked around for a bit before having a final drink at a hotel lobby bar near Madison Park and then hopped on the subway and eventually headed to our respective homes. Overall, we had a really great time and I looked forward to meeting up again.

During our first date, Matt shared that he and his wife, Terry, had been in an open relationship for almost their entire 15 years of marriage. Consequently, they had a lot of experience and comfort with navigating polyamorous relationships.

Along these lines, for our second date, Matt invited me to visit his home in Queens, which included the opportunity to meet Terry. I was admittedly nervous to meet her, but I was equally excited at the prospect. I also got to meet Terry's boyfriend. It was such a stark contrast to the secretive nature of what had happened with Dash and Dahlia and I was thankful for the experience.

Entering the Lion's Gate

I was learning so much in the space of a year. I was exploring my turn-ons and turn-offs, locating my desire and arousal, identifying and breaking old habits and struggling to overcome shame.

As I contemplated the intense shame and negative feelings associated with my sexual experience with Robert during college, I still felt so angry and defiled. I was still unwilling to name it as rape because I never said no, but I really didn't want to have had sex with him. Having had such a traumatic experience at that young age, there was a part of me that didn't feel safe or trust myself to know what I did or didn't want when it came to sex. I still didn't fully understand what had happened at that moment. Why hadn't I said no? Why hadn't I tried to leave? And yet, none of it mattered. It had happened and I couldn't undo the past; I could only move forward and heal.

So, as I worked closely with a sex coach, examining this trauma, I vowed to myself — to my pussy — that she could absolutely trust me to protect her from that point forward. And I truly meant it!

In early August, I had a first date with Lawrence, which I had been very much looking forward to since our initial connection on the dating app. We arranged to meet in his neighborhood. But it wasn't until I arrived at the restaurant and saw him coming down the stoop of the apartment building next door that I realized just how close to home it was. But, as I had joked with him earlier, I was happy to come to the East Village and thanked him for not living in Queens or Brooklyn.

We immediately hit it off and jumped right into deep conversation, sharing stories and otherwise showing ourselves to one another. He also revealed that his birthday was the next day, which meant that he was astrologically a Leo. I had remembered that August 8 was 8-8, the Lion's Gate, and explained the significance of this important date to him.

After dinner and drinks, Lawrence asked if I would come back to his apartment with him. I felt comfortable to say yes but made it clear that there was to be no expectation of sex. He readily agreed and we headed next door. I admittedly thought that we would start by sitting on the couch, talking and then kissing, but almost immediately we were on his bed, kissing and beginning to disrobe.

I was thrown off kilter as this wasn't what I had planned, and I wasn't sure what I did or didn't want to happen. I wasn't sure if I was ready or interested in engaging so physically with someone I had just met, no matter how exciting and intense the chemistry was.

Lawrence could tell that I was hesitant to proceed and gave me the space to share with him what I was feeling. I explained what was going on in my head and my need to slow things down considerably. He happily consented and we mostly just talked, kissed and held each other, clothed only in panties and briefs.

About an hour or so later, things began to escalate again, but it was infused with mutual want. He asked me to touch his cock, which I happily obliged, becoming wet with desire. He naturally felt into my lust and began to explore my pussy, checking in that I was okay and comfortable with his intimate touch. I most definitely was. He then asked if I wanted him, which I very much did, as long as he had a condom. He quickly put one on and then eased himself into me.

We proceeded to have sex, changing positions and really connecting. It was incredibly orgasmic, and it was obvious that we were both enjoying ourselves. I couldn't believe how good it was, especially given that we had only met in person a few hours before. Eventually, I needed a break and also realized how late it had gotten and decided to head home.

As I got ready to leave, I poorly paraphrased the expression: Start as you mean to finish, in reference to the intensity and intimacy of our first date. Lawrence was unfamiliar with the phrase but liked it as a harbinger of our budding connection.

I headed home on a high, still feeling all of the endorphins of my encounter with Lawrence, which I then shared with Viktor in beautiful, sensual detail until we were both sufficiently aroused to enjoy our own sexual liaison.

The next day, I noticed that a friend had posted an article about the Lion's Gate on Facebook and shared it with Lawrence. And it included this sentence: "Start as you mean to go on!"

The article further noted,
"August 8th marks the peak of an influx of high-frequency energy, onto planet Earth... It's a day that's been revered for thousands of years — as far back as Mayan times, this cosmic gateway has been marked on calendars and celebrated with ceremonies and ritual... Since ancient times, the Star Sirius has been known as the "Spiritual Sun". As the second brightest star in the sky (the first is our Sun) Sirius emits an energy that is hugely activating for us. Its light works to spur on the awakening process, it pushes us further into higher consciousness, and towards ascension."[9]

In the week that followed, I felt the power and the rush of having truly trusted myself. I had followed my authentic pleasure and desire. After many years of putting myself in unsafe situations and not protecting myself or my pussy, I was, instead, able to truly trust myself! I found myself standing at the Lion's Gate, with a higher consciousness and ascension.

---

[9] Please see: https://numerologist.com/astrology/lions-gate-portal/

In the wake of my incredible experience with Lawrence, I began to reflect on all that had happened. It was hard to believe that more than a year had gone by since that first, fateful party, catapulting Viktor and me into a new chapter of our lives. When we first decided to pursue this journey, we knew that it would be a positive experience, but that really didn't sufficiently capture the profound impact that this year had had on us as a couple and on me and my sexual awakening.

Almost ten years earlier, I had served as the anonymous interviewee (Charlotte – #5) for an article on sexual frequency in marriage in *Self Magazine*[10]. At the time, we admitted to having sex about once a month, but in reality, I think it was even less. And, this was after 13 years of marriage, which had been undersexed from the very beginning. I was shut down sexually; filled with shame, a lack of libido, and a general sense that wives (aka good girls) weren't sexual beings. Rationally, I knew that these thoughts didn't make sense, but I didn't know how to overcome their negative influence.

Thankfully, despite the lack of intercourse, we still remained close with shared intimacy — kissing, cuddling, hugs and a sense of being loved. This was never at issue or in doubt. Thus, I was eager to share my story in the magazine to let other women know that they weren't alone. But, while I was somewhat at peace with where things stood in my marriage and sex life, I knew I wanted so much more. It had been a lengthy journey, which was still unfolding.

It had indeed been a long road getting to where I was now. As the article mentioned, I had started my pole dancing classes as a way to explore my sensuality and sexuality and had found some benefit, but I knew it was only the beginning.

Through S Factor, I began to step more boldly and confidently into my body and, into my sensuality and sexuality. I began to own that I was, indeed, a sexual being. I still had to push past feelings of shame, but over time, I became more comfortable in that ownership.

---

[10] Beil, Laura. "Are You Having Enough Sex?" *Self Magazine*, August 2010.

My next conscious step on this path was enrolling in Mama Gena's School of the Womanly Arts. With its emphasis on women's empowerment from a place of pleasure, I had started to explore my body more intimately, making self-pleasure a more regular practice and learning to stay more embodied. This course of study and its concurrent immersion into an amazing community of like-minded women, was so beneficial as I continued to release shame and identify my sexual desires.

Yet, while I had healed so much, something was still missing. Viktor and I had greatly increased our intimacy, but our sex life still stalled from time to time. It wasn't until we chose to explore an open marriage that things shifted as seismically as they had.

Interestingly, for years, I had a recurrent, intrusive visual of a snake entering my vaginal canal and traveling upward and out my mouth. While I knew that this wasn't anatomically possible, I continued to have this unwanted image pop in my mind from time and time and finally shared it with my photographer during our pre-boudoir photo shoot session. She explained that this vision was very connected to Kundalini energy, but neither of us necessarily understood why I had continued to have this vision.

In the wake of all that had happened in the past year, I was convinced that this experience had finally awakened and activated my Kundalini energy that had been stuck and stagnant all this time. For the first time in my life, my body was responding in an intensely sexual way after decades of being shut down and non-responsive.

With each experience and encounter, I had learned so much about my body and myself, as I took the time to reflect and savor each moment. I had a long list of "accomplishments" such as performing on the pole, dancing at an erotic party, increasing the frequency of sex with Viktor, enjoying a threesome, having had sex at a sex party and being comfortable to walk around nude.

But, most importantly, I had gotten much clearer on my turns-ons and desires; learned about my body and its ability to climax in numerous ways; increased my intimacy with Viktor (and improved our marriage); increased my libido; increased confidence in myself and my body; met some incredible people; released shame; found my voice again; and learned to truly trust myself.

Moreover, this journey had come in waves, each one bringing its own sense of wonder, challenge and change. I was still a work in progress, but I was so excited about this personal transformation in achieving my lifelong goal of being a sexually alive being, capable of such pleasure and power.

As we arrived at our "Polyversary[11]" I wrote a love letter to Viktor.

My Dearest Viktor,

Wow! I can't believe that this past year has flown by. It has been such an amazing experience to go on this polyamorous journey with you as we pushed, prodded and pulled our marriage in new and exciting ways. Even more unbelievable is how much this has brought us closer together, increased our intimacy and dramatically improved our sex lives!

Early on in our marriage, when I was convinced that I was "broken," you stood by your conviction that you would rather be with me without sex than be with someone else with lots of sex. I even encouraged you to find a mistress, but you chose not to pursue this option. Instead, we found ways to maintain our connection and bond, but it was frustrating for both of us as we endured an undersexed marriage.

Despite this mutual frustration, we continued to thrive as a couple and I always knew I had your unwavering support whether it was my pursuit of S Factor and Mama Gena's School of the Womanly Arts or me dragging you to participate in a Tantra class, a D/s workshop, and enrolling us in Jaiya's program. No matter what, you always jumped in with both feet!

So, I knew that when I came to you with the idea of an open marriage way back in 2014, you would be willing to hear me out. You listened with an open heart and an open mind and, as we continued to revisit the topic from time to time,

---

[11] Polyversary was my made-up holiday celebrating our one-year anniversary of having had an open marriage, which dated to that first erotic party on May 4, 2018.

I felt even more sure that this was the right path for us to take, as we discussed what such an arrangement might look or feel like.

Regardless, I was just so thrilled to be having these conversations and so grateful to have made new friends who inspired me to question the status quo and consider a new paradigm for our sex lives. And you so lovingly welcomed Kimberly into our lives as we took baby steps in this direction.

Walking into that first erotic party last May without you was both exciting and terrifying. I had no idea what to expect or what might happen. Yet even though we hadn't expressly discussed anything, I knew I had your full support for whatever might occur. And your beautiful and loving response the next day, as I shared my experiences with you, reinforced that this was the moment we had been waiting for.

As the initial months of the summer progressed, it was clear that we had truly arrived at the Summer of Sexiness! Since that first fateful night, our individual and shared encounters have brought us closer, deepened my love for you, ignited my desire and opened me up to so much more.

With this first anniversary upon us, I want to thank you for having the courage to take this journey with me. Thank you for holding space when I needed it. Thank you for standing for me and my desire always. Thank you for standing for your own desires and sexuality. Thank you for being vulnerable. Thank you for being open. Thank you for your compersion and for your willingness to let me know when you felt less so. Thank you for your sense of humor. Thank you for your masculine and feminine energies. Thank you for your financial, emotional and physical support. Thank you for loving me despite my fuckups and maybe even loving me because of them as well.

Thank you for your unconditional love.

I know that we still have so much more to explore and learn, and I eagerly await this next chapter. I know that our love will continue to blossom and grow as we once again enter the Summer of Sexiness!

With love, lust and an open heart,

Jeannie

Part Three

I had thought that this story ended with my love letter to Viktor. We had had such an amazing journey up to this point and felt like we had accomplished so much. I had truly found a sexual awakening and finally achieved my goal of having a vital sex life with my husband!

Yet, while so much good had indeed happened, there was so much more to come that neither of us could have ever anticipated. We were about to be tested in ways that would push us, pull us and nearly tear us apart. Was our love and bond strong enough? We certainly thought so, but the next year was about to challenge everything we thought we knew about ourselves, about each other and about our marriage...

Shit just got real

Months earlier, Jon had sent me a link to a dating article[12] from *Ask Men* magazine. My first reaction to the article was that it was focused on Millennials who were unwilling to commit and thus didn't apply to us because 1) we had both committed via marriage to our respective spouses and 2) neither of us was a Millennial. I probed him further and he explained that he wanted to know if I thought there was a concern about either of us becoming attached to our relationship, revealing to me that he and his previous sexual partner had said (and meant), "I love you" to one another.

I re-read the article, which provided guidance on how to keep things casual in a relationship. Among his various recommendations, the author suggested limiting the frequency you see one another and avoiding romantic dates. Perhaps it was good advice, but I wondered... Which has greater influence on us: candlelight or cuddling?

Thus, I embarked on a quick Internet search, learning about chemistry and psychology. Science has shown that oxytocin, aka the cuddle chemical, which is released during intimacy, is a bonding agent

---

[12] Manley, Alex. "How to Make Casual Dating Work for You." *Ask Men*, April 25, 2019.

that makes us want to connect physically with another person and then stay connected. Along these lines, our pre-poly foray included a sexy encounter with our friend, Kimberly. She was averse to swapping spit (aka kissing) because she worried that I would become attached to her. I didn't think that a single night of passion could undo or hamper over 20 years of marriage, but I appreciated, and respected, her concerns.

Moreover, in the world of psychology, I discovered the concept of Attachment Theory (another foreshadowing of what was yet to come). First coined by psychologist John Bowlby, Attachment Theory refers to the emotional and physical attachment to another person that provides a sense of stability and security as part of one's personal development.

And, while Bowlby was primarily concerned with the successful social and emotional development of children, his ideas were extended to adult romantic relationships by Cindy Hazan (a professor at my alma mater, Cornell) and Phillip Shaver. And, of keen interest, Dr. Hazan's studies (and those of others) indicated "that people who have close social ties are happier and healthier and also live longer than people who lack such ties."

After a second read of the *Ask Men* article, I considered my relationship with Jon. While I didn't have crazy chemistry with him, I really did like him and enjoyed spending time with him. Plus, I felt somewhat connected to him as a result of what he had shared with me about his life, marriage, job search, etc.

Interestingly, due to travel commitments and hectic schedules, it was several weeks between the initial text conversation and when we finally saw each other in person. And then even more time went by after that meeting, which essentially became our last date. So, his concerns about love and falling in love were moot.

But, more importantly, as I initially reflected on the idea about becoming attached to someone other than Viktor, it didn't scare or worry me (at least in theory). I felt that as humans, we have a huge capacity to care about people. I believed that we could love multiple people without it negatively impacting any of those relationships in much the same way that parents of numerous children can love all of their children equally. Yet, all of these musings were theoretical and represented a relatively simplistic view of love.

So, at the time, I felt confident that I could develop feelings for someone else without it interfering with my relationship with Viktor. As long as Viktor remained my priority and my primary partner, I didn't anticipate any problems. Moreover, the strength of our bond and time invested in one another further reinforced my belief that a new relationship would be hard-pressed to replace what Viktor and I had.

Yet now that this idea of attachment had been broached, I was intrigued about what it might mean for these relationships that I was pursuing. Was there a danger of falling in love? Maybe. But I didn't think so. It was a bit naïve, but, at this point in my journey, the concept of NRE (new relationship energy) was completely foreign to me.

However, I did know that I wanted more emotional connections than simply having sex with different people, especially over time. I was becoming extremely dissatisfied with the flux and fluidity of the connections that came and went. I felt disposable as people continued to flit in and out of my life.

I knew I was so fortunate to have an amazing, loving relationship with Viktor, but I didn't think it was wrong to want more. In sharing this desire with Viktor, the idea was difficult for him, but I was confident that we would continue to discuss his concerns and allay any fears as we navigated this together, in a way that honored us both and our marriage.

But, what precisely did I mean when I said that it was possible to love more than one person at a time? Frankly, I am not sure I had fully thought it through, and it wasn't until months later that I realized that my view of love was much more limited in scope than those words indicated. The word love was one that would continue to trip us up time and time again.

In hindsight, we should have explored these ideas in more depth, pushing each other to be explicit in our definitions and desires. But we didn't see any danger signs, so we moved forward, and I began in earnest to find a "Boyfriend." Moreover, while I knew what I meant by this term, I wasn't sufficiently transparent with Viktor. I wish I had been more specific, but, as we have said, "You don't know, what you don't know."

Regardless of my (possibly poor) choice of terminology, I was eager to find an ongoing, more emotionally connected partner who made me feel wanted and special and wouldn't disappear after a few months.

In fact, with additional dating experiences — both positive and negative — I began to get a clearer understanding of what I genuinely wanted. My interactions with Eric proved that point in spades.

I generally go to my S Factor class on Wednesday nights and, on occasion, will schedule plans for after class. The first time I met Eric we had arranged just that.

Unfortunately, on my way to class, the subway decided to be very wonky going local (or as I like to call it, *slow*cal) instead of express. Thus, I arrived downtown way too late to make it in time. I was disappointed to miss class and texted Viktor about what had happened. He was sympathetic and invited me to meet up with him and his colleague for drinks at our favorite Champagne bar. I was able to join them for bubbles and light bites, having a fun time despite the frustration of not being in class.

At that point, I still had plans with Eric, but we had not arranged where to meet. I was feeling somewhat annoyed and contemplated canceling when he texted to say that he was running late and asked if 8:50 p.m. would work instead of our initial target of 8:30 p.m. Still on the fence, I consulted Viktor and his friend, and we all agreed that I would take a playful approach in my response.

I wrote back, "No, 8:50 doesn't work, only 8:52, but where?" He played along and let me name the place, so I told him to meet me at the Champagne bar. The three of us then had a small window of time before Eric arrived, so we advised our favorite server about our poly status, cleared the table to make it look like I had just arrived, and I then waited alone for Eric to appear.

Admittedly, I was less enthusiastic about the date at that point, feeling less than taken care of due to the lateness and last-minute planning, but we ended up having a really great time even though Eric is not a sparkling wine fan. We enjoyed getting to know one another and then shared an Uber which first dropped him off at his hotel and then took me home safely.

A few weeks later, we had our second date. Eric took me to dinner and then we went back to his hotel room. He had already asked me out for a third date while we were at the restaurant and I felt good about things continuing. However, I think that I wanted to make it work more than I really felt something for him and ignored the signs that it wasn't really what I wanted.

In particular, I had been dismayed by his lack of correspondence in between making the initial date and actually meeting in person — a span of several weeks in what I frequently refer to as dental appointment syndrome — and although this was better between dates one and two, I still craved more interaction from him. I mentioned this to him as I kissed him goodbye after we had had sex and he promised he would be in touch more frequently.

However, two days passed before he reached out and his text was rather unenthusiastic: "I made it back to Cayman. I very much enjoyed Tuesday night." Um, dude, we had sex; you could be a little more enthusiastic and complimentary don't you think? Apparently not.

His next text asked if I wanted to "try out CheckMates" on our upcoming scheduled date. Hell no, I didn't want to go to a swingers' club on our third date! I clarified his intent: "Since Checkmates is a swingers' club, it seems that you want me to have sex with strangers and/or sex with you in public. Is that true?" He replied: "Sex with you certainly. Sex with others is up to you." This was definitely *not* the fun date I was expecting when he had asked if I was available for that

Saturday night. I advised that this proposed plan was of no interest and he noted we could skip it.

In hindsight, I should have ended things there, but I waited to see what he would suggest next. He then offered up a trip to his house in Sag Harbor, which sounded fun, but when I probed for more details, he shared that he wasn't coming back until Tuesday early afternoon and wrote, "I can put you on the Jitney." Again, I was not pleased. My interpretation was that he wanted to take me to his house, have a meal and sex and then dispose of me the next morning by putting me on a long bus ride back to the city. I declined the invitation and noted that I no longer felt that we were a good fit.

He asked for clarification, which I happily provided:

"Yes, I will try to explain why I feel that way. It is mostly a feeling, but essentially, I don't feel really wanted by you. Among various things, I had asked you to text me more frequently, and yet it was two days after we had sex that you texted me and even then, it was a lukewarm text. Then, after only two dates, you suggested that we go to Checkmates, which really felt icky. And, while going to Sag Harbor sounds fun, the idea of being put on the jitney when you are done with me makes me feel like I am being discarded."

He responded rather quickly, but instead of addressing my chief complaint: "I don't feel really wanted by you," he proceeded to explain to me why he did what he did. I called him out on his response, noting that I wanted emotional connection and support, not justifications or explanations. And, consequently, ended it.

As I continued in my journey, I was learning what I did (and didn't) want. Yes, Eric was very wealthy and the fantasy of going to visit him in the Cayman Islands someday was very appealing. But I deserved so much more — more respect, more passion, more emotional connection and more emotional intelligence. And, equally important, I *wanted* all of those things.

I was admittedly frustrated with myself for having ignored my intuition and pushing forward anyway. I really did feel used and discarded and it coincided with the intense shame spiral I was feeling during my emotional rollercoaster ride — the first of many to come. Yet, I realized with complete clarity that I preferred to walk away from Eric rather than accept his crumbs.

Interestingly, Lawrence resurfaced that same week. He texted out of the blue looking to rekindle our relationship after a hiatus of nearly two months. He seemed sincere in his approach, so I was open to hearing what he had to say. I had been disappointed when things ended so abruptly with him but had really felt good about him and his potential.

We had a candid conversation, but it was evident that while he was very apologetic about the lack of communication and the way things ended, all he was looking for was a play partner. I thanked him but let him know that I had moved beyond that, seeking a more emotionally invested connection.

So, Viktor and I continued on our respective journeys, attending various events and utilizing dating apps to find both individual and shared partners. I was growing impatient, exhausted and frustrated in my inability to find a boyfriend but tried to remain hopeful.

In early September 2019, Viktor and I both had first dates on the same night, and we planned on meeting up afterwards and heading home together. On the subway, we shared our respective stories and were both encouraging and happy for one another.

On this occasion, I had been out with Sam and Viktor had met up with Justina, who he had met through his music community. Both of our dates had seemed quite promising and, in fact, my initial connection with Sam proved to be quite exciting.

With regard to Sam, it had just been a simple introduction on OKCupid — complimenting my smile and wanting to know more about me — but it was enough, along with his profile, to match and begin chatting. Thus, Sam and I were soon in an engaging conversation that captured my attention. He also introduced me to his wife, Shana, as there was the potential for the three of us to connect.

Thus, Sam and I had scheduled our first date for post-work drinks, during which the dialog flowed easily, and the hours flew by. We reluctantly decided to say goodnight and ended the date with a brief kiss. He texted on his way home (always a good sign and my preference) and complimented the kiss.

On that first date, we had talked about deliberately taking things slowly since I was looking for a more substantial connection to which he agreed. But, apparently, my kiss kindled something intense in him since the next morning he shared a very erotic dream he had had of me. And then the sexting began...in earnest.

Concurrently, Sam wanted to start planning date number two and even asked me out for the next night to the Philharmonic, but unfortunately those plans didn't work out. We instead settled on meeting up the following week, when I joined him and his wife for dinner at their home.

Over the course of the two weeks between our first and second dates, the sexting had been incredibly robust. His missives would ignite my desire and I would become wet thinking about him and what he was proposing to do to me. On occasion, it would fuel me to self-pleasure, and he was similarly fantasizing about me to ramp up his own at home sessions.

Finally, our second date arrived. I really enjoyed meeting Shana in person as we ordered in sushi, drank lots of sake and had a great time. However, despite all of us getting along, it was clear that this was a party for two. Eventually, Shana headed off to bed, as Sam and I sat on their balcony kissing and exploring each other's bodies.

A while later, we returned indoors and claimed the couch, feverishly undressing one another, anxious to have even more access to our sensual selves. It was hard (pun intended) to resist, but we remained true to our decision to not have penetrative sex, but it was delicious torture as he slid his erect cock over my clitoris, bringing me higher and higher. I encouraged him to come, which he did.

Two days after our date, we were texting and savoring the details of our time together. He had texted as he stroked himself to climax earlier in the day, but now it was my turn. I continued to type back my growing desire while grabbing two vibrators (one internal and one external). I alternated between self-pleasuring and typing until I came. It was an incredible experience to share.

Our third date was planned for a Friday night, two weeks hence. We were very much looking forward to having the time to truly get to know one another as well as take immense pleasure in each other more leisurely and at length since we would be at my apartment and Viktor would be at a rave until late.

One Tuesday afternoon about a week and a half before date number three, I decided to draw myself a bubble bath, bringing the phone with me as Sam and I continued our texting. He noted that he had to drive past my apartment on his way home from work, so I jokingly told him to stop by. Sam replied that if he did, then he would have to fuck me. I responded, "So?"

Not surprisingly, he happily obliged with a quick, post-work visit. He called briefly before he arrived and asked what I was wearing. "Bubbles," I answered, as I was still in the bath. Sam was only a few minutes away, so I quickly jumped out of the tub, toweled dry and draped on my robe.

Once I welcomed him into my apartment, we dispensed with a tour and headed straight to the guest room. It was a bit fast and furious, but we were so ready for one another after all of the teasing and texting. Yes, it was rushed, but it felt really good and I was enjoying the release of all that pent-up energy, eager to explore him more slowly the next week.

Unfortunately, it was supposed to be a prelude to the following week's date, but due to illness, Sam had to cancel our plans. He promised to make it up to me.

As this heated sexual energy continued to swirl around me, Viktor and Justina continued to build their relationship, texting back and forth over the weeks that followed.

One Friday night after a date with a new guy (which never went anywhere), I arrived home to find Viktor still awake. I filled him in on my evening and we talked about various topics.

Eventually, we started discussing Justina. I was happy to hear about how well things were progressing with Viktor and Justina and was excited about their new relationship until...

In a somewhat casual, off-handed way, Viktor revealed that he was in love with Justina. I felt like I had literally just been punched in the gut. It was such a visceral response. Wait, what? You just started dating two weeks ago and you are already in love with her? It hurt like hell and I began to cry. A steady trail of tears began to fall down my face; I felt fear and sadness and a host of other unnamed emotions.

I really felt badly about my reaction, which (in my naïve belief) should have been more positive and happier for him if I truly felt compersion, which I believed I did. But I wasn't going to deny my true feelings either. I was upset for myself. I wondered if I was still special if he could have such intense feelings for her so soon.

We discussed everything and Viktor apologized for blind sighting me and not being more sensitive to how he introduced the topic. He thought I already knew and was simply stating it again. I didn't, but I accepted his apology.

After talking through my emotional crisis, we came to a good conclusion and went to bed. I felt better the next day, but a week on, I was still raw and vulnerable as I continued to process the intensely painful feelings.

I questioned myself:
Did I have compersion? Yes
Did I have some jealousy? Yes

But I surmised that there was also envy and fear. Envy. How did Viktor get a girlfriend before I got a boyfriend? And fear. Does Viktor have sufficient love to share? I said yes, but did I honestly believe it?

Deep down, I knew that I trusted Viktor and felt certain that our bond was unshakable. I believed that our friendship and love endured and could withstand anything. The allure of Justina, their new relationship and what she brought to Viktor were deserving of Viktor's love and interest, but I felt that they wouldn't overtake or overshadow the love he had for me.

In a certain way, Viktor had gone from 0 to 100 in 60 seconds and I hadn't had time to adjust to seeing him with others more casually and then building over a period of time. But, like all of our various new experiences, I believed that it would simply take time for me to ease into this new status quo.

I was convinced that this pain was just a momentary blip and willed myself to move on from these negative emotions. I looked forward to getting to know Justina better, confident that time would heal my wounds, make me stronger and give me the wisdom to open my heart still further. This was what I had asked for; this was what I had wanted; and now I just had to be patient as I learned how to live in this new place. But there was no denying it, this shit was real! It was the first time this journey had started to challenge our marriage.

After that evening, Viktor's revelation continued to hit me hard. It took me several weeks to process the intense emotions that had been unleashed. I was very confused as to what I was specifically feeling and struggled to determine if I truly felt compersion for my partner despite saying that I did.

It hurt...a lot, and I wanted to make sense of everything so I could understand it and move forward and heal. On top of all of this, I was grappling with the loss of Sam. We had initially been texting three to four times a day with the added intensity of our sexting, which then dwindled to an occasional text every few days. What was up?

I missed the interaction with Sam, not just the fun, flirty, sexual innuendo (and the more overt conversations), but also the contact and budding friendship. Of course, I created all sorts of scenarios to explain Sam's telephonic absence and tried in vain to stop thinking about him. I felt the loss acutely, which felt even more painful in light of Justina and Viktor's blossoming romance. I felt lonely and a bit lost.

I vacillated between the two poles of pain, both equally unwelcome, as Viktor and I headed out of town for our anniversary. During that weekend getaway, we bared our souls, our bodies and our hearts, leaving nothing unexamined or unsaid. At last, I spoke my truth: I was afraid that Viktor would leave me for Justina. And, in exploring envy and jealousy, it became clear that I was deeply and fully jealous (fear!) as well as envious that Viktor had a girlfriend when I had only had a series of play partners. I wanted more.

But could I handle more? Sam's departure, finally confirmed at the airport post-weekend, left me uncertain on that score. If his exit from my life at this early stage could induce such painful feelings, what if I did truly fall in love with someone?

Yet my uncertainty with Viktor had been dispelled thanks to our candid conversations, intimate encounters and close connection all weekend. I left Miami feeling surer of our love and marital bond than ever. I felt my heart had opened and softened as compersion flowed more easily and with abundance. We returned home in great spirits.

With the amazing energy of our weekend away buzzing inside me, I started the week on a high. I was in love with Viktor. I was happy for him and Justina.

And then everything fell apart.

That Wednesday, Viktor and Justina had their first BDSM scene and sex date. I spent the evening at my dance class and then out with a friend, coming home cold, wet and miserable. Viktor had said that the door to the guest room might be open, beckoning and welcoming me to join them. But when I arrived home, the door was firmly shut. I felt it slammed in my face even though it hadn't moved or made a sound.

I removed my wet clothes, put on warm, cozy pajamas and crawled into bed, too upset to really cry. Viktor came to me sometime later and I desperately wanted him to stay with me — to choose me — but I felt too selfish to ask and I sent him back to Justina...sleeping alone and waking alone.

I awoke the next day feeling miserable. And I remained miserable for the next four days. I couldn't get over it. I couldn't stop the pain. I felt the shame spiral spinning out of control, coupled with agony and heartbreak.

I felt discarded, used and unloved. I couldn't stop comparing the superficial nature of my dating relationships — seeing them as cheap and tawdry through a cloudy and distorted lens — with that of Viktor and Justina's intense love connection. The pain of seeing him with her in my mind's eye, making love to her; it was unbearable.

I spent most of a Saturday curled up in bed on one long crying jag before I eventually fell asleep for the day. Then the rest of the weekend found me on a roller coaster of emotion soaring from intense heights of self-hatred to extreme lows of depression; I almost wished I were dead, but I was not going to act on such intrusive, negative thoughts.

A big part of me wanted to simply put an end to the open marriage, but I was truly trying to be fair and balanced to Viktor. I hated the way I was feeling both in terms of the pain but also its impact on him. This was not my intention, but I needed to protect myself and my sanity.

Throughout that weekend, we continued to talk, keeping our options open, knowing that I was not in my right mind to make any major decisions at the moment. We agreed to take it one step at a time — helping me to heal and make sense of what had happened and why it hurt so damned much. After that, who knew? I just knew that we would get to the other side of this together and had no doubt that we would come out even stronger.

Yes, I was confident that we would get to the other side of this together, even stronger, but I wasn't to know that this was only the beginning of an intense saga that would have me vacillating between euphoria and angst, on a constant roller coaster ride that would last for a very long time.

Hit hard by Viktor's revelation that he was in love with Justina, it was a deep dive into depression, with many crying jags and endless discussions that truly threw me for a loop. But, eventually, I knew it was time to pick myself up and dust myself off, knowing that this painful place wasn't where I wanted to be.

I hated the selfish nature of what I was feeling and was very conscious about not derailing Viktor and Justina's new-found relationship. Yes, I was struggling with jealousy, envy, shame and doubt, but I knew that I needed to allow these emotions to move through my body if I was ever going to heal and move past them.

I welcomed the sadness and the rage, nearly drowning in them, but also using these deep, dark emotions to call in the love and support I needed from my sisterhood community. I shared my feelings in safe forums and was held with loving arms as I mired in the muck and mud of the figurative swamp. Those aware of my situation reached out via text to check in and offered kind words and just generally let me know they were there for me as needed.

I also contacted two friends who had much more polyamorous experience for advice and perspective. For one of them, the idea of Viktor's being in love with Justina would have been a violation of the rules she and her partner had. Yet, she didn't judge; she merely lovingly offered me a number of things to consider with respect to the agreements I had with Viktor and the current situation with Justina. Another friend talked about how he wasn't wired for compersion and suggested that I might not be either. I was grateful to both for their candor and willingness to share their wisdom with me.

In addition, I knew that it was important to strengthen my relationship with Justina and invited her to meet with me. She readily agreed and we had a genial lunch on a Friday afternoon. While we spent a lot of time just getting to know "fun facts" about each other, I made sure to address the elephant in the room.

Justina was aware of what I had been feeling through her conversations with Viktor, but I wanted to tell her in my own words. She was very willing to hear me out as well as modify her behavior as needed. I appreciated her offer and told her I would let her know if there was something that I wanted from her. I felt reassured by her respect for our marriage and assured her that I liked her and liked her for Viktor. I just needed to process this new experience for myself.

And throughout it all Viktor and I continued to talk. And talk. This was not for the faint of heart. It was challenging to tease out the tangle of emotions that this experience had thrown at me. It was difficult to determine how best to balance self-preservation with selflessness for one's partner. It was and would continue to be confusing to figure out my role now that I was no longer my husband's one and only.

Out of the darkness and into the light

With all this self-exploration, I continued to alchemize most (definitely not all) of my jealousy and negative emotions, at least for the time being. And, thankfully, this transmutation enabled compersion to flow more easily and freely. I generally felt good about Viktor and Justina, but I didn't pretend that it would be all smooth sailing from there on out.

In the wake of this most recent roller coaster ride, I had good days and even some really great days. And, yes, there were dark days, too. Seasonally, it was a tough time for me (I suffer from Seasonal Affective Disorder), so I was not at my full strength, but I coped as best I could and, I had no doubt that I would persevere and overcome the sadness. This was a work in progress and, like me, it was not perfect. But it was wrapped up in love and trust and beyond that, I simply needed to let go and feel into that trust...trusting myself, trusting love, trusting Viktor and trusting the universe.

Life continued on as it does and in early November, Justina, Viktor and I were scheduled to go to the House of Love party on Friday night. And, while I was a little nervous, I was very much looking forward to our first foray into the world as a polycule.

Our evening became a little more complicated when Gigi not only started dating Dan (who was then my employer as well as my friend), but also decided that they, too, would attend the House of Love party. We agreed to pregame with them as was our usual plan with Gigi pre-House of Love events.

In addition, friends Lane and Nolan who I had met on Feeld, but befriended instead of dated, had taken me up on my invitation and were excited, but anxious, to be at the party. Plus, my friend Kaya, who had had an unhappy experience at the previous House of Love party, was giving it another go. So, there would be a big group of us there together.

I made sure to head to the grocery store in advance of everyone's arrival at our apartment and set up all of the food and wines, wanting everything to look perfect for our guests. Eventually Justina, Gigi and Dan arrived, and we enjoyed light bites and drinks before finalizing our costumes and heading out.

Once we arrived and hit the dance floor, my inner "Julie McCoy, Cruise Director" kicked in. I felt very responsible for making sure that everyone was taken care of, watching out intently to find various friends and making sure they were all having a great time.

Seeing that Gigi and Dan were kissing, Viktor and Justina were dancing, and that Lane and Nolan were off somewhere, I accepted Kaya's invitation to go dance on the elevated platform, eager to be a good friend and to have somewhere to put my attention. We continued to dance together for about an hour or so and then went off to the flogging station for our respective scenes.

Once done, I knew that Viktor's volunteer shift (as a consent monitor for the event) had begun and I went off in search of him. I found him dancing with Justina and tentatively joined them. I felt like a third wheel. I didn't know how to behave or act. I was confused and felt a little left out, even though neither of them did anything specific to make me feel that way. I just wasn't sure where I fit in if I was not Viktor's only date.

A short while later, Justina was ready to head home and kissed Viktor goodbye. I averted my eyes and gave them some privacy. I was so *not* ready to watch my husband kiss someone else. Then, he and I remained on the dance floor, but I was overcome with sadness and a little FOMO of having been focused on everyone but myself. I had had a nice night, but not an awesome night and felt a little cheated.

Viktor and I continued to dance, rejoining with Kaya as well as with Lane and Nolan, as Viktor's volunteer shift ran for another hour and a half. At one point, Lane turned to me and asked if she could kiss me. I was very flattered by the invitation and happily consented. It was very sexy and exciting, but I knew that nothing would come of it beyond the dance floor, which was fine. By that point, she was first and foremost a friend, not a potential play partner.

Yet, even that delicious kiss couldn't fully pull me out of my funk and as we headed home in the cab, I allowed the tears to flow. It was initially tense because I knew Viktor was upset with me for being in a negative emotional state, but he was unaware as to why I felt the way I did. I gave him permission to feel whatever way he wished to feel but asked him to hold off on sharing his frustration with me in that moment. He agreed and, instead, reached out to comfort me and I let him.

As the tears eventually subsided, I was able to explain what I felt and why, giving Viktor insight and context, which helped him to better understand the state I was in. I felt extremely connected to him and felt his love and support.

We arrived home exhausted, but in a really great place, and fell asleep soon after getting into bed. The next morning, we continued our conversation, working through anything still left unsaid and allowing us to address all of our varied emotions. I felt particularly good about where things stood with Viktor and Justina as well as with Viktor and me. It hadn't been the most amazing House of Love event for me, but there was no doubt that my heart was filled with love.

After the weird House of Love party, I was confused. What was next and what did I really want to happen? I was just about to give up and take a break, but fortunately life had other plans, putting me back on track and back into my body.

I kicked off the week with a friend for happy hour, setting the stage for a great week to come. Then, on Tuesday night, Viktor and I had plans to go to a BDSM Party with Tova. I was so thrilled to be embarking on this journey with her, shepherding her exploration. We all set intentions on the subway there, putting forth three desires each. My desires were: 1) to stay awake (since I had been up since 3:00 a.m.);

2) to play in some way at the party; and 3) to interact and flirt with others.

As we walked into the venue, I was overcome with anxiety, but tried to push past it. We were immediately welcomed into the event and soon met a number of people, actively engaging in various conversations. I saw that Tova was taken care of as she talked at length with the event organizer and I knew that Viktor could fend for himself, so I relaxed and enjoyed meeting new people and observed a few kink scenes from the sidelines.

Once Tova decided that she was ready to engage in a rope scene with Viktor, I eagerly set a container for them and held space, mesmerized as I watched the two of them together. It was beautiful to witness, and I was so happy that she had such a positive first experience.

Just prior to their scene, one of the male guests had asked me to Dom him. I explained to him that while I was interested in stepping into this persona, I had extremely limited experience. He didn't mind and encouraged me to play with him. As Viktor and Tova were cuddling on the couch, I consented to be his mistress, negotiated the rules and set him on his tasks as my submissive.

I had him fetch drinks for Tova and Viktor and me and eventually had him compose a poem in ode to (as well as kiss) my thigh-high boots. It was fun, but also a lot of work and I wasn't sure what else to do with him. He kneeled nearby, but once it was clear that I was moving on to another play partner, I released him and thanked him for his services.

By this point, I had started talking with Austin, who had caught my eye upon our initial arrival at the party. Once I saw that he was doing a Shibari suspension, I very much wanted to play with him, especially since Viktor was too tired to do another rope scene after his time with Tova.

Austin and I negotiated our scene, and he began to tie me, binding my arms behind my back and ultimately secured me to a wooden post. He next moved on to more sensual pursuits, raking my naked skin with long, metal claws and ultimately kissing me. It was extremely erotic and alluring and I continued to enjoy his company as he held and kissed me during aftercare.

As we prepared to depart the party, I gave Austin my phone number and he texted me before I got home and again in the morning to check in on my well-being post-scene. Suitably intrigued, we scheduled a playdate for the coming week.

Still infused with the sexy energy of Tuesday night's event, I had a fun and fabulous first date with Trevor on Wednesday after my dance class. We met up for drinks and connected right away. I was pleasantly surprised to feel attraction and chemistry after the failure to feel these things with other recent first dates. It reinforced that I needed to trust myself better; if I was not attracted to someone's photo online, I was not going to feel attraction in person. Message received loud and clear!

During my date with Trevor, he noted that he liked to meet his partners' partners. Of course, I didn't think he meant on a first date. However, when he went to the restroom, I checked my phone and saw a text from Viktor that he and Tova were at a place nearby. Then, as I was responding to his text, they walked into the bar where I was and ultimately met Trevor when he returned! Thankfully, it all went well and, as I kissed Trevor goodbye, I felt really good about our date. Soon afterward, he asked me out for date number two.

With all of the positive encounters on Tuesday and Wednesday nights, by Thursday, I was in a wonderful mood and felt that the balance in our relationship had been restored. I felt buoyed by the flirtatious attention, dropping further into my body and simply feeling happy and content. This was the perfect place to be as I reconnected with Gary (the professional Dom), having a low-key scene with him on Thursday afternoon. I knew that I was back to my old self as my confidence and equanimity slowly returned.

Then, I wrapped up my amazing week on Friday with a duo of fun events. During the day, I met up with Nate at the Whitney Museum. This was our third date, and I was excited to see him.

Our first two dates had been on Wednesday nights after dance class and thus had been limited to drinks and light bites. While I had definitely enjoyed our first date, it wasn't until our second date that I had really felt the connection and potential. On date number two, Nate had inquired about what had been going on since our previous meeting and I asked him if he wanted the nice answer or the truth.

He responded that he wanted the truth, so I shared with him the reality of what I had been feeling ever since Viktor had started dating Justina. Nate had a long history in the poly community and was able to listen to my stories and hold space. Later in the evening, he shared a vulnerable moment with me. I could feel his beautiful, intense energy as he held my body against his and felt safe and seen. I knew I definitely wanted more time with him.

Thus, it was nice to have had a full day to spend with Nate and to get to know another side of him, since he had a lot of knowledge about, and experience with, art.

As we kissed goodbye after our day at the museum together, we expressed our desire to have more private time in the future and I eagerly awaited getting to know him more intimately. I was afraid to anticipate too much but was open to possibility.

That same night, I closed out the week with a return visit to House of Yes with Viktor. While it was a much tamer event than House of Love, it felt a little bit like a do-over from the week before and it was really nice to have him all to myself. We enjoyed an awesome performance from Little Boots before heading home, knowing that all was well in our lives once again.

For our first date outside of meeting at the BDSM party, Austin came over to our apartment for a scene. I was clear with him up front that I didn't know if I would want to have sex with him. He was okay with this, so we agreed to proceed. That evening, we had a four-hour scene with rope and sensual play, taking turns as Dom/Mistress and sub. Things did become very physical, but I deliberately chose not to engage in penetrative sex because I didn't really know him, and I wasn't sure where things were going with us. Would we see each other beyond this evening?

I was still unsure what I wanted to happen on our second date but knew that I wanted to get to know him better. Thus, I requested a non-scene date. He offered to cook me dinner and invited me to go to a paint and sip event near his apartment.

We had a lovely dinner and then snuggled and kissed for a bit afterwards before heading to the art event. We then returned to his apartment and got cozy on his bed. Things progressed with time and we were eventually both naked and enjoying each other's bodies, but I told him that I wasn't sure I wanted to have sex. As we continued to tease and turn each other on, I began to have an in-depth conversation in my head.

The central question for me was whether to have (or not to have) sex with Austin. It should have been a simple question with a simple answer: yes or no. Yet, it was far from simple. I wondered whether we would see each other after that night. Did I want that? What did I want from him? For us? Would this become a one-night stand after he got what he wanted, aka sex? Would he stop calling and texting? Did he care about me or was it just sex?

I worried that this most recent encounter would become just another name added to the list. I didn't want to inadvertently create a lengthy list of men I had had sex with. All of this turmoil pointed toward saying no. This was a situation fraught with lots of uncertainty and I wasn't sure how having sex would be a favorable decision amidst all of it.

Concurrently, another part of my brain thought that saying yes to sex was just easier. There was the ease of his climax versus giving him a handjob or oral sex. There was the ease of repayment for dinner and the event (I had only paid for the wine). In general, it was just easier to skip ahead, zone out and just give in. I had knowingly turned him on, he clearly wanted to have sex (he stated it verbally) and on and on. So, why not? Why not simply say yes and have sex with him? Of course, I knew that these were stupid, pointless arguments, but they streamed through my mind anyway.

It was a two-sided argument with only one participant and despite all of the rhetoric and discussion points, none of the conversation addressed the real question: Did I *want* to have sex?

Thankfully, I was eventually able to turn off my mind. I waited and felt into what I was *feeling*, not *thinking*. And, what I felt was Austin's energy. I felt aroused. I felt alive. I felt wanted. I felt desired. And I realized that I desired him. I truly wanted to have sex. So, I said yes, enthusiastically!

I trusted my body to tell me what I wanted, and it was a deliciously orgasmic experience. I felt really good about my decision afterward and had no regrets or remorse about it.

Meanwhile, Tim and Nate had gone radio silent and I wondered if they were still interested in dating me. I made up scenarios in my head as to why they weren't getting in touch.

While I would be disappointed if those connections had run their course, I wanted to know. I wanted the closure. So, I used a technique to "locate" where they were in regard to me and our respective relationships. I texted each of them, indicating that it seemed that they weren't interested in pursuing our respective relationship and asked, "Is that true?" They each texted back within 48 hours, confirming their continued interest in me.

Nate readily acknowledged his lack of communication and explained that he was going through a rough time and didn't want to seem like he was complaining. As a result, he had said nothing. Meanwhile, my head had concocted a story that his monogamous primary partner was having issues with him dating others and therefore he didn't want to see me anymore. In fact, he revealed that he had been thinking of me every day.

Clearly, there was a need for better, more ongoing communication in all relationships. I understood and respected privacy, but it was so helpful and necessary to just send a quick text to let someone know what is going on.

Along these lines, I was most appreciative when Gary reached out to tell me that he was dealing with some personal issues and needed to go dark for a while. Simple, yet effective. I felt valued and respected and, in turn, respected his need for space. He later told me that it had taken him 30 minutes to craft the text, but I assured him that his time and effort had been well worth it.

As these experiences showed me, no matter where we were in a relationship, we needed to have clear and open communication with our partners — and with ourselves. And when it was an issue of feeling instead of thinking, we needed to know how to trust ourselves and navigate that conversation as well. Anything else was just a waste of time and energy.

The pain of pleasure

Things were reasonably good for a while. I was pleased with what I was learning about myself and with my ability to locate and communicate. However, over a period of several weeks, I wasn't able to move beyond my own pain to focus on Viktor's pleasure. Instead, I was feeling quite miserable and had even been suicidal for a short time.

Some of this could be attributed to my compulsion to find a boyfriend. I am admittedly single minded when I have something I want and often approach things with a "to do" list mentality. Accordingly, ever since I had decided that I wanted a boyfriend (and even more so in the wake of Justina's arrival), I had been actively pursuing this goal. Yet, unlike "Buy bread" or "Pick up dry cleaning," it was not as easily checked off my list.

One week, I had the not-so-bright idea to schedule five first dates within a single week, with the expectation that at least one would work out. My intention was to schedule as many dates as possible and to schedule them close together so I could compare and contrast them, believing that their proximity to one another would provide greater clarity in knowing who/what I wanted. In the end, it was an exercise in futility and frustration. Honestly, it was too much, too soon and too tiring. So, despite my diligence, my agenda item remained unaccomplished.

The following week, things continued to be incredibly difficult for me. I thought I was finally in a really good place about Justina and Viktor, but then Viktor took his friend Avalon to a BDSM party and they became play partners.

Compared to a girlfriend, this should have been easy for me. Yet it was still so hard. First off, when I got home after their play date, there was some confusion between Viktor and me because I thought I was going to have dinner with them, but due to various reasons, it didn't work out and I felt left out. Also, they were in the den eating and watching TV, which was not a welcoming setting compared to if they had been sitting at the dining table.

That being said, the other, more important, thing was that, again, this wasn't simply a sexual connection. In fact, at this point, I was not sure if Viktor was capable of such a thing. He knew Avalon from the music community in which he was so immersed, so they already had a strong energetic connection before sex was introduced.

I had already been jealous of the time he spent in this community and, for the majority of the time we had been open, had actually been focused on trying to find partners who were available on Friday and Saturday nights, since I was spending so many of those nights home alone while he was out at raves until the wee hours of the morning.

When Viktor shared his encounter with Avalon with me, instead of being turned on by it or happy for him, I had an intensely visceral, negative response; I screamed and began to hyperventilate. It was scary and uncomfortable. Even a few days later, it was still so raw and painful to talk about and I again started to breathe irregularly. I didn't want him to censor himself, but I couldn't change what I felt, no matter how much I wanted to.

And the three times I had been in the same room with her, she had hugged (or had attempted to hug) me without my consent, which was offensive and uncomfortable to me. I didn't know why she thought I would want any contact from her — physical or otherwise. Did she think I wanted to be friends? She was fucking my husband; I was never going to be friends with her.

Further, as I reflected on what had been coming up for me emotionally, I realized that for me, sexual intimacy didn't mean that much on its own; it was just sex. But true emotional intimacy was sacred to me. I could only share that with Viktor. The fact that he could share it with others hurt like hell and made me feel shut out. I knew he loved me, but if he could have such an intense bond with more than his lawfully wedded wife, where did I fit in anymore?

I wasn't sure what this meant going forward. I was trying to stay open (both literally and figuratively), and not close out Viktor's activities because I didn't want to be unfair or be hypocritical, although we agreed that we were not precisely comparing apples to apples.

I was also reexamining my interest and motivation for being polyamorous. When we first began this journey, it was all about finding my sexual turn-on and desire. I didn't know why it had taken such an unconventional approach to do so, but I had found it in abundance and was so thankful for the experience and for having gotten to this place in my sexual awakening.

But I no longer thought that having multiple partners was necessary for this particular aspect of my journey. I thought that I could continue to find my desire with Viktor alone. I was not making any snap decisions, but I was simply trying to figure out what made sense for me and our marriage.

In the meantime, I said goodbye to Austin because, at 28, he was a child (or at least acted like one: living with three roommates, without a guest towel in the bathroom and exhibiting juvenile behavior) and I deserved a man.

I was still seeing Trevor and Nate but was not sure if either of those relationships was going anywhere. Neither of them liked to maintain ongoing contact and there were long stretches of time between texts and making plans. As it was, I had only had four dates with Nate even though we first connected in late September and it was now

December. I had had only marginally more interactions with Trevor in a slightly shorter timeframe. I felt like I was waiting around to be remembered, which didn't feel good; I wanted to feel wanted and desired.

Going forward, Viktor and I continued to talk openly as we headed into the new year, exploring opportunities, reconsidering rules and boundaries and overall choosing what was best for us.

We also spent a lot of time talking about finding new ways to spend more time together. More specifically we hoped to explore new interests and activities that included, rather than excluded, me. Over the past few years, Viktor's music community had become particularly important to him and very time consuming and immersive. I didn't begrudge him for getting so involved on the surface, but I had begun to feel very left out of his life even before we opened up our marriage. This new focus sought to bring us back to each other and was an equally important discovery as we evaluated our situation.

As we welcomed the new year and new decade, I tried to put my dark emotions behind me. Admittedly, the Fall and Winter had been much more challenging for me on this journey compared to the lightness I had experienced much of the previous year. As Mama Gena says, I had been playing *all* 88 keys (perhaps especially the sharps and flats). But, despite these negative experiences, I still believed that this journey continued to be a positive one for me *and for us*. Thus, I felt a renewed buoyancy as we slowly shifted from the nadir of the Winter Solstice and once more welcomed the sun's return.

On that note, I was confident that Viktor and I were poised for great things in the year to come. I was encouraged by the amazing conversations and communication that we had had over several weeks. Yes, they had been difficult, if not downright painful, but we were yet again increasing our intimacy and strengthening our marital bond. I had no doubt that our marriage — and our love for one another — was stronger than ever.

Moreover, I was feeling excited about his relationship with Justina as it continued to ebb and flow, evolving with time to become what they both wanted and needed from each other. And I was hopeful about some of the potential relationships that I was courting.

In truth, I had a lot of irons in the fire and was waiting to see which one would be forged into the relationship that I truly desired. Along these lines, Trevor and Nate were both still in the picture and I was enjoying their company, unsure what would or wouldn't happen with either, both or neither of them.

Consequently, I had a fun overnight date with Trevor that provided me with the opportunity to pole dance for him, which was lots of fun, despite accidentally kicking him in the shin (oops!). Meanwhile, Nate and I had not yet ventured beyond kissing, but he had expressed interest in a play date so I was hopeful it would be scheduled in the next few weeks. Unfortunately, Gary had inexplicably ghosted, so I no longer had a Dom to explore with, which was disappointing (and confusing).

In the meantime, Viktor and I were finding our footing with respect to Avalon. I tried to remain open but had come to accept that I just didn't like her and was perfectly justified in feeling that way (in that I had no obligation otherwise), thus freeing myself up from unneeded angst and allowing me to stop expending energy in that direction. Moreover, our conversations surrounding their relationship put me at ease, permitting me to move on without malice or fear.

Another bright spot in our journey was a play party with Playscapes. We had attended their mixer back in December in anticipation of the next play party. At that event, we met Connor with whom I had an immediate and intense connection. In the weeks that followed, we had occasionally texted each other and looked forward to connecting more physically at the event.

Once Viktor and I arrived at the play party, Connor and I quickly found each other. I really liked his sexual energy and felt amazingly comfortable in his presence. On an interesting side note, it turned out that Austin was also at the party, but it was nice to see him, without any discomfort or drama on either end.

A short while later, Connor invited me to go to the playroom with him, which I happily accepted. As we talked and kissed, we were joined by Viktor. The three of us slowly engaged in play as Viktor tied a Shibari harness on my chest, easing me into the sex scene. I was admittedly nervous since I had only played full on at a play party once before and it was with the help of edibles. On this occasion, I was resolved to be fully present and clear headed and deliberately abstained.

Once we got going with kissing, touching and undressing, it felt powerful and heady to have both of their attentions directed at me. I was very aroused as was Viktor and the two of us were soon having penetrative sex, which was very enjoyable. I then hoped to have penetrative sex with Connor, but he had a little bit of performance anxiety, so we took a short break. Eventually I had sex again with Viktor, climaxing intensely, which was a very pleasant surprise given the public nature of the event. Somehow, I was able to block out the "noise" of others around us and just focus on the pleasurable sensations of being with the two men.

A while later, we decided to get dressed and return to the bar area for drinks. During this time, Connor noted that his previous play party experiences had all been with couples, so I thought that he might enjoy the opportunity to have some alone time with me. I asked Viktor if that would be okay with him; he agreed and departed.

I sought out Connor and advised him that if he wanted me all to himself, he could have me. He eagerly consented and we returned to the playroom, disrobed and were soon having sex, which was a lot of fun, bringing us both to climax. We were then rejoined by Viktor, who had been watching from afar. At this point, Connor excused himself (and ultimately left to head home as it was getting quite late), while Viktor and I had sex again before calling it quits, ending on a high note as Viktor exploded in a beautiful, energetic orgasm.

Being surrounded by sexy sounds and scenes was very intoxicating to both of us and made us realize that we crave to play again and engage with more people. We looked forward to integrating this new piece of information as we further discovered our sexual interests and desires.

Poly-Anna has left the building

When this journey first started, it was all rainbows and unicorns, but the latter part of the journey was filled with many ups and downs, so my outlook became decidedly less rosy. Instead, things had become more challenging as we maneuvered the complexities of being in a polyamorous relationship.

Our initial foray focused on a simple opening up of the marriage, with ethical non-monogamy, but no expectation of emotional attachments. Then, Jon mentioned the idea of falling in love, which prompted a series of conversations with Viktor and sparked my desire to find a boyfriend. I observed that the situation seemed to work well for two of the men I had dated, who each had a wife and girlfriend (in addition to me).

I also thought such an arrangement would eliminate the never-ending flux of situationships, which left me feeling, at best, like a revolving door, and, more often, abandoned for a myriad of unknown reasons as many (not all) men behaved very badly.

At almost two years in, Viktor had such an arrangement with Justina and, while it was a little less intense than at first, it was no less emotionally connected than when he first told me he was in love with her. In addition to him being in love with her and loving her, they planned lots of dates in advance and texted on and off in between dates. And, because they were both active in the music scene, they often saw each other at events, even if it wasn't a scheduled date.

In truth, I was at least a little happy for them. I envied what they had, but I no longer felt intense jealousy because I trusted Justina and Viktor and I didn't fear that she was a threat to me or our relationship in any way. Yet, I still felt like crap, a lot of the time.

Some of that had to do with the fact that I had been actively trying to find a boyfriend since August of the previous year, but without success. This fruitless search left me feeling bereft at times; occasionally less than and even unwanted. Yes, I knew that my worth had nothing to do with anyone else, but it was hard to not take such things personally sometimes.

Given all of the angst associated with my dating life, a big part of me wanted to simply give up and stop. But another part of me felt that I would not feel whole again until I had balance; me having a boyfriend to balance out the fact that Viktor had a girlfriend.

While I knew that Viktor didn't love Justina more than me, I had begun to feel that he loved me less than he used to. I didn't actually *think* he did, but I definitely *felt* that he did. We talked about this at length and he promised to do better to make me feel more loved and to know that I came first. But, I wondered, if we have an abundant supply of love to give, why did it feel so scarce?

And, while I knew it didn't make any sense, I somehow felt that I needed to find someone to replace the love that Viktor had taken from me. I think this was what had pushed me to be so focused in my approach to dating. Logically, I knew that Viktor's love should be sufficient. Moreover, I intuitively knew that I needed to fill my own tank with self-care, sleep, self-pleasure and self-love. But, in the meantime, I still felt the loss none-the-less.

As a result, I really struggled with whether or not I wanted to continue to pursue a poly lifestyle. The intricacies of full-blown, emotional relationships could be rewarding (I thought), but at what cost to my emotional health? As I thought about it, it was difficult for me to simply date to enjoy the journey; I felt driven to succeed in my goal. Could I step back and re-frame, reassess and reclaim the fun? I wanted to.

I wanted to be able to savor what I had in the here and now and not worry about what would or wouldn't develop. Easier said than done (at least for me). The relatively safer path of open (but not poly) beckoned, but I was not yet decided.

As had been our practice throughout this adventure, Viktor and I continued to talk and evaluate where we were and what we wanted. I was cautiously optimistic but would wait and see. The scales had fallen from my eyes and I was no longer a Pollyanna; I had not yet left the building, but I was definitely eyeing the exits.

Men behaving badly

This disillusionment was further exacerbated by the departure of various men. While I realized that my dating experiences echoed what a lot of other women go through — I was not alone in being brushed off and ignored — yet I felt it so viscerally. It felt like an abandonment and I didn't understand the behavior.

I truly couldn't fathom why it seemed to be so difficult for people (in this case, men) to simply state their truth: I have changed my mind/I am no longer interested in pursuing this/etc. While I might not be thrilled to receive such a message, it was much better than no message at all. And it was certainly better than being ignored.

Admittedly, the ghosting wasn't new, but, as I had shifted my dating focus from dating for sex to dating for connection, it felt more hurtful, especially as timelines had grown longer. In particular, my first date with Nate took place in late September and was followed by two more widely spread-out dates in the fall. He seemed to disappear at one point, so I reached out with my locating spell: It seems like... (in this case, that he was no longer interested in dating me). He immediately wrote back and apologized for his radio silence, citing health issues. I gave him the benefit of the doubt and asked him to be more communicative, noting that he didn't have to share anything he didn't want to share, but just to let me know that he was busy or otherwise distracted. He agreed and I thought we were back on track.

After the December holidays, we arranged to have an overnight date at his house in New Jersey. On the day of our date, Nate drove into the city to pick me up and, during the car ride to his house, we had a heart-to-heart talk, during which I asked him to kindly text me back within two days of my texts to him and to make plans with me in advance, rather than waiting until the last minute, since I was likely to already have plans. He readily agreed and we went on to have what I thought was an amazing date.

On the way to his house, he kindly stopped at the grocery store to pick up cheese and crackers and breakfast for the next day. Then, once we arrived, we hung out talking/ dancing/kissing in front of a roaring fire all night, finally heading to bed at 5:00 a.m. In the morning, he made us breakfast and then drove me back into the city, reaffirming his commitment to plan in advance and communicate in a timely manner. I was optimistic and excited about where I thought things were headed.

Yet, two weeks went by without a response to my text or a request to make a date. Really? I sent another, less gentle text questioning his inability to meet my requests, and then, a week later when there was still no reply, gently asked for an explanation as to what had happened. I never heard from him again. But I was truly at a loss to understand the situation. This guy was interested enough to continue dating me for four months and yet, he decided to ghost after all of that (and especially after an epic, sexy date)? WTF?

Less egregious was Trevor, whose texts became fewer and farther between. I knew that he had some family health issues going on and simply sent supportive texts in his direction, but eventually noted that he was sending mixed messages, i.e., asking me to meet him for drinks one night and then recanting and telling me he had to work.

While I respected his need to work, I did wonder if his enthusiasm had waned and questioned him on it. He finally wrote back to say that yes, he was now interested in finding a primary partner, but hadn't wanted to hurt me. I sincerely thanked him for his honesty because really that was all that I wanted. Yes, I was disappointed to see him depart, but I wasn't overly invested in him and I also wanted him to find what he desired. If that wasn't me, so be it. But, if I hadn't pushed, I am fairly certain he would have ghosted as well.

Lastly and perhaps, most hurtful, was Gary, the professional Dom I had been seeing since July of the previous year. Things with Gary had been going well, with us meeting up about twice each month. He had become a D/s mentor to me, permitting me to explore various kinks in a safe and sane way, which I greatly appreciated.

Moreover, he had presented me with a collar in late September as a reward and recognition of what our relationship had become. It meant so much to me and it seemed to be meaningful to him as well. While our dates were mostly centered on D/s play and sex, he had invited me to see an off-Broadway show with him and had spent a lot of time really getting at my interests and desires within the kink scene.

Our last date was in early November and an additional meet up was forthcoming, during which time he said he would send me possible dates. I never received any dates and followed up with a text. No response. I didn't want to push too hard and gave him space over the holidays, but even a well-crafted submissive text requesting an explanation yielded no response, leaving me feeling used and discarded. He was free to change his mind about me, of course, but I had placed a trust in him as my Dom that he broke. I think that in his position of power, he had a duty of care owed to me that he completely ignored. In the aftermath of that, it was challenging to believe anything that was said or done in that context.

So, yes, I felt that these men had indeed behaved quite badly. It was not that time consuming to send a simple goodbye text. And at least two of these three men knew how I felt about ghosting and yet they did it anyway.

Ghosting seems to be the new normal, but we shouldn't accept it or make excuses for it. What happened to decency and respect? If you had been physically intimate with someone (read: sex), didn't you owe them the time and energy to end the relationship in a respectful manner? At a minimum, I was perplexed, but, more to the point, I was hurt and admittedly afraid. I knew it wasn't fair to judge someone based on the poor behavior of others, but I was finding it difficult to trust as I proceeded with dating.

Thankfully, the men I was currently dating seemed to be capable of kindness and respect and I was hopeful that whatever happened with those relationships, they would provide me with examples of men behaving much better, thereby restoring my trust and dispelling my fears.

Some like it (red) haute

As February 2020 arrived, I mused, "Could I reclaim the fun of this journey?" Fortunately, the answer was a resounding "Yes!"

It had been a difficult and emotional week. In addition to feeling lonely and much less loved, I had also had a heated discussion with Viktor on that Thursday night. Of course, feeling less connected to one's partner was never good, but it felt especially vulnerable in the run up to Valentine's Day. Thankfully, by the conclusion of our intense conversation, I was more at ease with the situation and ready for the holiday.

For Valentine's Day, we had decided to go to the House of Love party at House of Yes with Gigi. Given the event's coincidence with the holiday, the theme was Red Haute. Despite planning my costume for weeks, the morning of Valentine's Day, I was less excited about this year's plans because last year had been so amazing. Plus, my last venture to House of Love had not been a great success, so I had some trepidation about what the night would bring. Time would tell...

In spite of a less than enthusiastic outlook, I headed into my Friday with an upbeat attitude, which was well rewarded. My usual Friday S Factor class was great, and I had an awesome dance, unlocking new emotions and finding new movement.

After class, I returned home and mulled over my conversation with Viktor from the night before, which had centered on my use of dating apps. He felt that I should consider getting off of them for a while and, as I thought more about it, agreed that it would be a healthier and less goal-oriented approach for me to limit myself to meeting people in person.

As I set about deleting Fetlife, OKCupid and Feeld, I messaged any existing matches and advised them to contact me via kik if they were still interested in staying in touch. Within a short period of time, I heard back from Dylan, the male half of a couple with whom we had an upcoming date. Dylan and I had a fun and flirty exchange of texts, which fueled my energy and infused me with feeling sexy and excited for Gigi's arrival for our usual House of Love pregame of wine and cheese.

Suitably dressed and made up (Gigi had done Viktor's makeup), we headed to the event. In the car heading to the venue, we set our intentions and desires for the night ahead. Mine included kissing at least someone other than Viktor, having fun, feeling sexy and confident, relaxing into the night, and not having my feet hurt from dancing in my new shoes.

Once we were settled at House of Yes, we decided to wait in line for the photo booth. While awaiting our turn, we saw some friends and also met a couple who were interested in hearing our poly/open relationship story. As Viktor and I talked honestly to the woman, her male partner spoke to Gigi. Somehow, he was under the mistaken impression that Gigi was Viktor's girlfriend and asked her, "Do you ever feel left out?" Gigi had no idea what he was talking about and it was, at first, a confusing, and then, amusing, discussion once the oversight was corrected.

Photos taken, we headed to the dance floor. Viktor and I had made the commitment to really enjoy Valentine's Day together and because I was feeling more in need of attention and love, we had agreed that he would be less focused on finding others and that the night would be more about me. We stuck to this plan and it worked out beautifully.

At some point during the night, Viktor had to step away and I was dancing on my own. Shortly thereafter, I was approached by a guy whose name was Ari. He asked me if I was there with anyone. I told him I was there with my husband but expressed my desire to dance with him.

Apparently, he had other plans than dancing. Instead, he said, "I need to get you a drink," took me by the hand and started pulling me, but we were headed in the opposite direction from the bar. Oh, perhaps we were going to the bar in the other room? But wait, no he was taking me to one of the VIP areas! He made me a drink and proceeded to compliment me and kissed me. He told me how attracted he was to me — heady compliments for sure — and then said, "My girlfriend will love you."

Truly intrigued (this night was getting even more interesting), I replied, "Well then, I'd love to meet her." Ari left to go find his girlfriend wherever she was and left me in the VIP area for quite some time. I was beginning to think he had forgotten about me when a guy entered our section and introduced himself as Adam. He asked me where I was from. I explained that Ari had brought me, but he was more interested in knowing where I had grown up, etc.

Adam and I proceeded to get to know one another and were soon kissing. Then Ari returned very briefly, kissed me and then disappeared again. Admittedly, neither Ari, nor Adam, were particularly consent-oriented, but, in the moment, I trusted myself and chose the role of pleasure researcher rather than that of consent monitor. Moreover, it was not the most conducive environment for a teaching moment.

Ari returned, this time with a woman named Nina (not his girlfriend) and Ari, Nina and I shared a joint kiss, before Ari headed back out to the dance floor once again. Adam, Nina and I talked for a bit, and soon Adam was kissing Nina and then pausing to kiss me. After some time, Nina departed, leaving Adam and I to ourselves to continue kissing and eventually more.

Amidst all of this, Ari appeared and introduced me to his girlfriend Brittany with whom I shared a brief kiss. There was then a flurry of sexy activity with handjobs, blowjob requests (which I emphatically declined), breast fondling and a drooling incident (as he was kissing me, Ari drooled/spit on me. Gross; I told him to never do that again!). Ari invited me to come home with him and Brittany, but I demurred.

I eventually decided to take my leave of Adam and Ari and return to Viktor and Gigi, both of whom I easily found on the dance floor. We continued to enjoy ourselves as we danced late into the night, departing House of Yes at 4:15 a.m. Viktor and I arrived home at 5:00 a.m. and began to enjoy some intimacy; it had been a week since we had had sex and we were excited to be with one another, especially since it was Valentine's Day.

Suddenly, the phone rang. Who was calling at this hour? It was Gigi and she was locked out of her apartment. We immediately invited her to come over and spend the night in our guest room. While we awaited her arrival, we knew that we had about 15 minutes, so we resumed having sex and were able to finish quite pleasurably before she appeared at our door. It was a pretty amazing quickie! We then got Gigi settled into in the guestroom, excited to have an impromptu slumber party.

The next morning (or rather, three scant hours of sleep later), Viktor and I woke up still feeling quite amorous and proceeded to have morning sex, which was super rare for us (mostly because it was rare for us both to be getting up at the same time). However, it proved to be super orgasmic and we were both blissfully spent by the time Gigi was awake. Then, Viktor made us all breakfast, which turned out to be such a fun way to continue the energy of the night before. Overall, it was an epic night filled with sexy vibes and had definitely been red haute!

Between a rock and a hard place

Despite the fun and festive nature of our night out at House of Love, I was still in a very dark place as I mulled over our polyamorous status. I continued to struggle with everything that was going on and, on top of it, Viktor had some very real other emotional issues that he was dealing with. Going to him with my painful feelings just wasn't an option.

Viktor and I had been talking a lot lately, trying to make sense of things. But I felt like things between us were not yet resolved and I felt very anxious about it. Moreover, a particular conversation shed light on some rather disturbing truths.

The first was when Viktor noted that he had called Justina to have "another shoulder to cry on." It really hurt to know that he was reaching out to her in his time of need. Reaching out to her for advice made sense but knowing that he needed her comfort and support made me feel really uncomfortable.

The other, more pressing concern was our repeated discussions centered on closing our marriage. From the very beginning, we had always said that if one of us wanted to end our open status, we would immediately do so. Any time that I had considered such a decision, I had always promised Viktor that I would give him some time from decision to actual closure. This made sense to me and gave me the feeling that if things went south, we could always go back to the way things were before we had opened up our marriage.

Yet, one night in February, Viktor said that while he would abide by my potential decision to close our marriage, he would be left with resentment and anger. This was completely unexpected. Moreover, he asked to continue to be friends with Justina and even possibly continue their BDSM relationship. I said, maybe, but upon further reflection, I was so *not* okay with this.

Such an arrangement felt like Viktor would be adhering to the letter of the law, but not the spirit of it. He wouldn't really stop being polyamorous, he would simply stop having sex with his partner (with whom he didn't have that much sex anyway). I didn't want to tell him who he could or couldn't be friends with, but I didn't see how it helped us go forward, if things didn't actually change. It wasn't the sex that bothered me as much as the deep emotional attachment, which was the whole point of considering the closure.

It seemed like our two options were:
Jeannie being unhappy
OR
Viktor being unhappy

I didn't know how to reconcile these two things.

I did know that I didn't want to lose Viktor and I didn't want to jeopardize our marriage.

Or was it actually:
Jeannie being unhappy
AND
Viktor being unhappy

If I condoned us having a poly relationship, I was condemning myself to more misery, but if I made the decision to return to monogamy, I could very well lose my husband due to anger, resentment and continued attachments to outsiders. I truly didn't know what to do.

With my successful burlesque performance in late February, I had a brief respite. But early March was yet another low point for me. We were supposed to go to a ropes conference with Justina and all I wanted to do was die, to simply fade from the picture and cede Viktor to her. I couldn't go on. Moreover, I kept thinking we could end things, but each time I felt Viktor's reluctance to say goodbye to Justina. Their love was too enmeshed; he loved her too much to live without her and he resisted my pleas. I could sense that I was truly between a rock and a hard place.

Our repeated discussions on closing our marriage left me confused and scared. Uncertain how best to proceed, I relinquished control and continued to go on with the status quo despite my pain. I martyred myself in service to Viktor and Justina, suffering in silence.

In one way, nothing Viktor had done (by loving Justina) was wrong and yet I felt the shift in our bond so viscerally in my body, namely in my chest, like tiny daggers digging their way into my heart; wounds from which I slowly bled. I tolerated the pain; I tolerated his love for her; I tolerated the situation; but at what cost to me and our marriage? This wasn't what I had anticipated when we opened up our marriage in search of a sexual awakening. For me, it had all been about lust, not love.

The trouble with trauma

By early spring, the cracks began to show as I saw what all of this dating had been doing to me. It was making me anxious, unhappy, feeling used and abused, etc. I was unable to let go of the goal to find someone and, now that I knew that I wanted a boyfriend (and was no longer dating for sex, as I had been initially), I was even more worried about dating because I feared that I would end up with even more ghosting situations that would leave me feeling worse.

I was so thankful and grateful for the sexual awakening that this journey had brought me, but I was so fucking fed up with all of the angst, anxiety, depression and other negative emotions that it had brought as well.

In sharing my pain with our friend Tova at the time, she listened closely and noted that it very much sounded like I had abandonment issues and asked some questions about my mom. As I reflected on what she said, I was in full agreement that the conditional nature of my mother's love had indeed been a source of early trauma that was likely being triggered now with all of the dating departures. The repeated withdrawal of her love in those moments in which I had displeased her were so painful and had felt like I had been abandoned by her again and again, leaving their mark. I read several related articles that resonated very strongly and reinforced what Tova had suggested.

I also did some reading on how such abandonment issues might impact someone in a polyamorous relationship, wondering if such trauma and polyamory could co-exist. The short answer was: No.

As Maria Merloni, MSW noted on her blog, "To keep it really simple: abandonment issues + polyamory = disaster."[13] Yes, of course, it's an oversimplification, but as Roan Coughtry wrote,

"Fears of abandonment are real and very common — especially when you've been abandoned in the past by someone you love. This fear can be so deeply wired that no matter how much reassurance or affirmation you get from your partners, lovers and comets, you may still find yourself waiting for the other shoe to drop. Polyamory can especially bring up fears of being replaced, although these fears can exist in monogamous relationships too."[14]

This knowledge, and subsequent self-diagnosis, was quite startling, yet very revealing, as my anxiety and fears suddenly made much more sense. This didn't make it any easier to cope in the short-term, but I

---

[13] Merloni, MSW, Maria. Abandonment Issues and Polyamory. *Maria Merloni.com*

[14] Coughtry, Ryan. "Guest Columnist Roan Coughtry tackles a reader's polyamorous abandonment issues!" *I am Poly and So Can You.* May 23, 2019.

was acknowledging and owning my past trauma and recognizing how it was impacting me currently.

Journaling in early March 2020, I wrote,

"I feel so stuck. Now that I know that my anxiety and fear are caused by deep-seated abandonment issues, I feel both good and bad. It's good to be able to pinpoint and identify the root cause, but it seems exhausting and overwhelming to overcome this obstacle... I feel unloved and unworthy of love. I can't see beyond past hurts and disappointments. I can't believe that I am truly loveable."

Yet, I started to take responsibility for my self-healing and investigated various treatment modalities and options to get well in the hope that this path toward better mental health would help me become more comfortable with the poly lifestyle and alleviate some of the pain it was causing me. I knew it was a long road ahead, but, while I felt stuck, I was also hopeful, now that I had a better understanding of myself.

An incredibly difficult two weeks followed, as I struggled to make sense of where we were on this journey and how I was feeling about it. Mercury in Retrograde and continued Seasonal Affective Disorder all conspired to make me even more emotional than usual. Consequently, I was on a rollercoaster of emotions yet again, driving Viktor (and likely others) understandably nuts, but throughout we remained connected in our communication, no matter how painful or difficult.

I did a ton of Googling (and subsequent reading) on various poly topics in an attempt to better understand what this all meant for Viktor and me. We hadn't exactly planned for all of that to happen — it just sort of did — and were then dealing with the consequences, not all of which were bad, but all were new.

I had fallen in love with Viktor at 17 and I didn't think I had ever stopped being in love with him despite dating others in between that tender age and getting married at 26. I was still very much in love with him and genuinely believed that he was my soulmate.

For over 20 years, we had been just the two of us. Now that it was the three of us, it felt as if everything that I knew and believed had changed. I wrestled with figuring out how we could still be soulmates if he had room in his heart to fall for someone else. There seemed to be divided views on this topic in the polyamorous community, but, at least to some, the two were not at odds. I took heart in that.

On the flip side, it felt so foreign to me to think that I could ever love anyone else in a romantic way. Yes, I love my close friends, but that was a different kind of love. I just didn't know if I could find room in my heart for anyone new in that way, but I was trying to remain open to the possibility.

After being Viktor's wife for nearly 25 years, I wondered what sharing this role with others indicated as to who I was. What was left for me that set me apart as special and sacred? I knew that there was so much more to our love than this implied, but it was challenging to embrace these changes after all this time. And it was hard not to feel competition for limited resources.

I was definitely pressing edges on all sides, trying to learn to expand my definitions and overcome ingrained behaviors and beliefs. I was also in the midst of processing old traumas and was at the start of what appeared to be a long journey of healing and recovery. It hurt. A lot. But I was confident that I would prevail.

Fortunately, as I contemplated the road ahead, I knew that I was so blessed to have the love and support of my friends and community. This had been a tremendous help to me in staying as grounded as possible despite being on a ship adrift in the high seas. I felt special gratitude to Tova for having been my land-based skipper as our boat sailed ahead on this uncharted voyage.

After the turmoil of a two-week period, I finally began to feel that I could breathe deeply again. My nervous system felt more at peace as I worked to let go of the fight or flight response that had plagued my body and mind for months. I was optimistic that Viktor and I would weather this storm as we had done with all of the others — hand in hand. Together. Always.

I felt much more grounded, happier and calmer. I still had moments of doubt, but I felt stronger and was more easily able to push these adverse thoughts away. I also felt more connected to Viktor as a result of this tumultuous period. It wasn't my preferred way to increase intimacy, but I gladly took the positive outcome to what was otherwise a very negative experience.

As I looked to further bolster my mental and emotional health, I actively sought out external guidance. As much as Viktor and I continued to talk and kept our lines of communication open, it felt like time to reach out for help. I was hopeful that such outside exploration would permit me to become clearer on what I truly desired for myself and for our marriage, as well as permit me to release hurt and pain more effectively.

Concurrently, we also began to consider couples counseling, scheduling consultations with a few therapists, so that we could benefit from the perspective of a trained professional. Someone without a vested interest in the outcome, other than our collective well-being. We were committed to making this work, both individually and together. But before we could schedule our first appointment, the world fell apart with the arrival of the global pandemic.

Soon afterward, there was no money for therapy on a joint or individual basis. The world was on lockdown until further notice...

Part Four

It was the best of times, it was the worst of times

S o life as we knew it was (at least temporarily) closed for
business. These were unprecedented times, and we had no
way of knowing when (if?) the world would return to its
regularly scheduled programming. Until then, we found new
ways of doing, behaving and communicating. Thankfully, we had the
benefit of technology to assist with some of this, although I found that
a return to low/no tech was a welcome change.

Those first few weeks of the crisis pushed some people together
and pulled others apart, as we self-isolated and social distanced. I was
exceedingly grateful that Viktor and I weathered the storm together
from the comfort of our shared home, along with our pup. Prior to the
cocooning, we had already been taking the time to really talk through
our feelings and concerns in a calm and measured manner (in direct
opposition to many of our heated altercations).

The weekend right before lockdown included a three-plus hour
discussion that covered every topic at least once and ensured that we
were in full agreement on how we viewed our marriage and how we
wanted to move forward on our poly journey. As a result, we felt
extremely close and connected to one another and love flowed easily
between us once again.

Amidst these conversations, we tried (mostly in vain) to identify
concrete definitions of love in its various guises. In an overly simplified
definition, I noted that, for me, loving a friend was taking care of their
cat while they are away even though I don't like cats whereas loving
someone romantically meant that I wanted to spend every waking
moment with them.

Admittedly, I didn't mean it quite literally, but the universe has a
great sense of humor! We knew that there would be challenges to
separate our mundane day-to-day life in close quarters from more
sacred connections to one another. We would have to be imaginative
with date nights given our limited activities and resources, but I knew

we were up to the challenge. Interestingly, we were pleasantly surprised by our attendance at a virtual orgy early on, proving that technology could offer some creative solutions to creating quasi-physical connection.

As we headed into the unexpected, I felt surprisingly calm. I felt that I had undergone such a profound transformation on many levels over the past few weeks leading up to lockdown. The early part of the year had found me in and out of a dark place as I teetered between intense highs and lows with regard to my marriage and poly life. I battled with myself and with Viktor, trying to overcome jealousy, envy and abandonment issues.

But, as Viktor and I had been able to enhance our communication, clear the air, get clarity on our mutual desires and generally reconnect with one another during this time, it had strengthened our bond and confirmed that we appeared to be on the same page. Consequently, it had instilled a renewed sense of security and safety in me. I was in a good place emotionally and mentally despite the pandemic.

Conversely, we were separated from our other partners. I knew that it was hard for Viktor to not see Justina in person. They texted frequently and had video chats and movie dates via Netflix Party.

For my part, a relationship begun in earnest in early January waned, while a more nascent relationship took an interesting turn of events. Just prior to the pandemic, I had made the commitment to eschew dating apps in favor of in-person events and thus, one Wednesday night in early March, I found myself at a poly mixer at which I met Alex.

Before quarantine, we had exactly one in-person date. Since that first date, we had been texting back and forth. A lot. We had intense physical chemistry from our initial meeting that carried through to our in-person date and then into our written communication. We enjoyed flirting with one another and were also having fun sharing memories, desires and just generally getting to know one another. Plus, we shared the love language of Words of Affirmation, further fueling our sexy banter.

This on-going correspondence felt old-fashioned in a really sweet way and also served as a novel approach to building deep emotional connection in the absence of physical contact. Alex further upped the stakes, sending me an exceedingly romantic love letter. Swoon! I really loved the bond we were creating with one another through this mutual exchange.

A few weeks into our courtship, we had an hour-long phone call, which was the first phone call I had had since I started dating. It was luxurious to hear his voice, share our thoughts on BDSM and other sexual matters and simply revel in having each other's undivided, synchronous attention. While we were both anxious to see each other, we knew that our eventual in-person meet up would be all the better for having had this time to connect emotionally and personally.

Over the next few weeks, Alex and I continued to deepen our connection as we progressed in our beautiful relationship. We had cemented our emotional bond more firmly through exquisite texts and poetry, while concurrently fanning the flames of desire with our "lust letters" to one another. It was quite heady and deliciously arousing. I was pleasantly surprised by how close I felt to him and how much he turned me on from/despite the distance and lack of in-person contact.

By April, we were happily reaping the benefits of the slower pace of work and life and really enjoyed the opportunity to deeply connect with one another.

By that point, our dates had included our single, face-to-face date at a wine bar (during which there was a lot of face-to-face as I eagerly kissed him again and again), an hour-long phone call and two video chats. At this rate, we anticipated that our second, in-person date would coincide with our six-month anniversary!

Our first video chat was relatively straightforward, but for our fourth date, we sought to recreate physical intimacy via virtual tools. I had tossed out the "totally crazy" idea of doing a mutual, self-pleasure session and Alex readily agreed.

Of course, while we were both excited about the prospect, we were equally nervous and anxious. In anticipation of the call, I realized that the level of intimacy on which we were about to embark was perhaps greater than if we were actually having sex.

I felt so vulnerable and more figuratively naked in sharing this experience with Alex. And yet, because we had developed such a strong emotional connection, I completely trusted him to move forward with it, choosing to disregard the butterflies in my stomach.

In preparation for our time together, I pretended that I was getting ready for a real date. I took a shower, shaved, sprayed on perfume, styled my hair and donned a sexy set of lingerie. I also surrounded myself with LED candles and a glass of wine to suitably set the mood, as I waited to connect with Alex on Zoom from the comfort of our guest room bed.

Once online, we spent time talking and connecting. Alex had the lovely idea to take turns and ask each other questions about our respective self-pleasure practices. It was a fun way to slowly slip into the right frame of mind while also getting to know each other better. We then switched to a game of Truth or Dare, which essentially became a back and forth "dare," encouraging the other to remove one article of clothing after another until we were both fully naked. So far, so good.

The last set of dares upped the ante as Alex dared me to turn on my vibrator and begin to pleasure myself and I dared him to stroke his hard cock. We accepted each other's challenges, continued to talk briefly and then I knocked back a shot of Tequila, took a deep breath and proceeded to really focus on my self-pleasure while Alex watched from afar, further fueling his own turn-on.

I came quite close to a full climax, but eventually stopped. I was a little self-conscious of the time I was taking, knowing that I had an audience and couldn't provide physical touch and reassurance the way I would during a usual, in-person intimate encounter.

Then, I switched my focus from me to him, as I watched Alex bring himself to orgasm. It was an incredibly sexy experience, sharing such an intimate moment with him. And, truly, even better than I had expected when I had hatched this preposterous plan.

Post virtual coitus, we spent a little more time talking and then wished each other good night. A short while later, I joined Viktor, who had been watching a live stream with various DJs all night. Not surprisingly, he had heard my climactic moans and screams from the other room and was quite turned on. Still extremely aroused from my interactions with Alex, I was equally interested in physical play with Viktor. He pulled me to the couch and entered me as I simultaneously stimulated myself with the vibrator, heightening my pleasure and eventually exploding in an extremely intense, blended orgasm.

Fully sated, I tried to head to sleep, but was way too wired in spite of the late hour. As I laid awake, I replayed my time with Alex in my head, realizing that this was definitely not something that I could do with just anyone. It really required a high level of trust, connection and a willingness to be extremely vulnerable. But I was immeasurably grateful to have shared this encounter with Alex and to have added to the intimacy of our relationship.

Love and lust in the time of Coronavirus

As we went into week six of social distancing, like everyone else, we had our share of good days and bad days, neutral days and a few "I am so fucking over this" days. Through it all, we continued to nurture various relationships, including our own. And, while in some cases this was easier done than in others, we were committed to building connections in their various forms and functions.

Along these lines, my relationship with Alex continued to blossom. We texted each other multiple times a day, often sexy texts, sometimes silly ones and always communication that brought us closer together. It had been amazing to see how we were building a deep emotional connection, while sustaining the intense chemistry we first felt at our initial meeting — all through technology. We had our weekly video chats that included physical intimacy that, while virtual, was also very real and authentic. I had struggled with trying to name, define or quantify our relationship, but eventually gave up, realizing that labels did not matter; what we knew that we felt for each other did.

Rather, I let go of fear and embraced the possibility of love in all its guises. If this period of isolation had taught me anything it was that life was too short to be afraid. So, I stood on the edge of an emotional cliff, ready and willing to fall, daring to dream, and believing that what was meant to be would be.

After spending nearly four months in a virtual relationship, or perhaps more accurately, developing a relationship at a distance, Alex and I finally had our second IRL date. We had planned the date weeks in advance to coincide with his return to New York (he and his wife had spent a month in South Carolina) and in collaboration with Viktor's date with his Friend With Benefits to ensure we would have the intimacy and privacy we desperately craved.

Alex was due to arrive at our apartment at 8:00 p.m. I took the day off from work, enjoyed pampering and primping myself at leisure and baked muffins in anticipation of our breakfast the following day. Once dressed and mostly ready, I met up with Gigi in the park for a sunset happy hour.

Gigi and I lost track of time and Alex was a little earlier than expected, so a few minutes before eight, the Intercom rang on my phone indicating that Alex was at the front door...and I was still at the park. Oops!

I apologized, told him that I would be there in two minutes and ran down the street and into his arms, upon arrival in front of my building. It was so amazing to be in his arms after all that time apart.

We reluctantly disengaged long enough to open the door and enter the apartment before I flung off my mask and began to kiss him. I was thrilled to discover that I had not imagined our chemistry or how good it felt to simply kiss him.

We paused briefly to open some wine but were soon kissing again as Alex scooped me into his arms and carried me to the guest room. He was like water to me — I had been parched as if in the desert; he was quenching my thirst for him as we kissed and held each other for a long time.

Then, I began to undress him and slipped out of my dress. We took turns removing each other's underwear until we were both blissfully naked. We continued to explore each other's bodies, which had previously only been available to us on a screen, mapping every part with our fingers and tongues. We were hungry to touch and learn after being denied this physical intimacy for so long. It felt so relaxed and natural to be together even while we were so eager to be with each other.

I was very aroused and very wet as Alex pleasured me with his fingers and mouth before I told him how much I wanted him. He then slipped on a condom and then slid into me, with both of us eventually reaching orgasm.

As I had predicted, there was an intensity and eagerness in our mutual inability to truly wait and slow down, yet it was equally infused with tenderness and humor. The magic of our reunion was sweet, sacred, sexy and all around perfect. We further reveled in the ability to simply be in stillness and silence with one another, freed from the need to talk, text or otherwise respond with words.

We continued our pursuit of pleasure with one another for several hours, then turned out the lights and went to sleep, nestled in each other's arms. The next morning, we happily awoke and resumed our sexual discovery.

We eventually pulled ourselves out of bed to get coffee and enjoy the muffins I had made. We lingered over breakfast before Alex got dressed and packed and I walked him to the subway entrance with a final kiss goodbye.

A short time earlier, with May's arrival, I had reflected upon Polyversary #2. Viktor and I celebrated our second polyversary with a quiet night at home (of course, it was still a pandemic after all) and a rope scene (our first in months). While it was hard to believe that another full year had passed, in truth it had been a particularly tough year.

The previous May had found me in high spirits ticking off a long list of amazing accomplishments from our first year in an open marriage. I was thrilled with how much our marriage had been strengthened and with how far I had traversed in my sexual awakening, overcoming so much sexual shutdown and shame. Viktor and I were in a fabulous place and we were poised for another great year.

Well, it wasn't the year that either of us anticipated, that's for certain. And, although I didn't relish the pain and suffering that I (and we) had endured, I was not sure that I would change anything.

It was a tempestuous season; we were blind sighted by a love neither of us expected and were not prepared to deal with. Yet we muddled through the trials, tribulations and a lot of tears to get to the other, brighter side of this storm. But though it all, our resolve to be together never wavered; we remained stalwart and steadfast to our partnership, believing in our destiny as soulmates and in the purity of our love.

I was grateful that Viktor and I had not only weathered the storms but came through them stronger than ever. We strengthened our bond and recommitted to our marriage and to one another while we also expanded our circle of love. Our communication skills had become laser sharp as we learned how to better handle the stress and strain in more constructive ways to get to resolution. We had reaffirmed our love and deepened our connection. And we knew that we loved each other — truly, madly, deeply — and were together because that was what we genuinely desired.

In looking back, it was a year of trust as I learned...
to trust myself and my body,
to trust our love,
to trust what Viktor said,
to trust my heart,
to trust my desires,
and to trust that I deserved love.

It was a year of discovery about the inadequacy of words and the way they fail us.

We say one thing, but is that what we really mean? What does our partner think we mean?

We struggled to understand the difference between envy and jealousy.

We tried to parse out meaning for ourselves and for each other when we talked about love and being in love. Was there an actual difference and what did that mean for our own love and relationship?

It was a year of searching...
for meaning,
for understanding,
and, yes, for a boyfriend.

It was a year of overcoming as I overcame fear and trauma. I dealt with abandonment issues. I had not overcome jealousy, but I had gotten better at dealing with it. I had no doubt that I would always be jealous in this regard, but it had been helpful to have my own, more secure relationships to balance out that loss.

That summer we were in a time outside of time; everything and nothing was possible all at the same time. It was during this period that I had somehow found myself in an improbable, yet exquisitely beautiful, relationship that was a beacon of hope in the darkness of despair and the fog of uncertainty.

Interestingly, as we acknowledged this milestone on our journey, I still didn't know what I wanted for the long-term. If this next year brought more heartbreak, I didn't think it would be worth the hardship, but for that moment, I had let go of labels, expectations and limitations and was just being, feeling, existing, experiencing.

And so, summer had arrived with a renewed sense of jubilance. Was it once again the Summer of Sexiness? Perhaps? As things with Alex continued to blossom and grow, I was so grateful to have him in my life and to see what we were developing together.

But it was short-lived. Despite the beautiful relationship that we were co-creating, underneath I was still deeply unhappy. And fighting with Viktor resumed in earnest. I felt his focus on Justina keenly as she dealt with various crises one after the other and he rushed in to save the day. Honorable? Yes. But it made me miserable.

The beginning of the end

At our wits end, by August it was clear that our situation was unsustainable on its own and we resumed our search for a poly-friendly therapist to help us out. By the end of the month, we had made the financial commitment to couples counseling despite the fact that Viktor had been out of work for five months; our marriage was too important.

While I tried to be open to whatever outcome, I harbored a not-so-secret fantasy that we would return to monogamy as it seemed like the only way to ease my continued pain.

What did I desire?
I desired closing our marriage.
I wanted my husband back.
I wanted peace of mind.
I wanted to be happy again.

Our therapist asked us to articulate our goals as well as to find our "why" with regard to having an open marriage. I felt I had lost the thread of why we were doing what we were doing other than the fact that Viktor loved Justina and I was holding onto Alex in a desperate attempt to feel whole and balanced. In truth, my connection with Alex was much more than that, but it was hard to keep that perspective sometimes.

We had developed a ritual of going to the nude beach on fair-weather Wednesdays and on one occasion wrote out our goals and also added objectives in support of those goals:

Goal: To re-establish our intimacy and relationship so that we both feel loved, whole, calm, connected, safe and secure; that heals our connection; provides a shared language and vocabulary; restores trust, and permits us to express our feelings without judgment and engage in productive communication with one another.

Objectives:

- Develop a shared understanding of what we each mean by the word love and develop a shared vocabulary so that emotional connections are clearly defined/understood.
- Define and determine our needs, wants, and desires as to what we want our relationship to look like in terms of monogamy/non-monogamy and create a contract or framework as applicable.
- Determine how best to manage feelings of jealousy and envy in a constructive way.
- Overcome past wounds and nurture each other in supportive ways that heal instead of hurt.

At least we had a roadmap for our counseling sessions and knew where we wanted to go. It would not be an easy road ahead.

We each had a reprieve with a lovely Labor Day Weekend in-person reunion with our respective partners, but by early fall, I was once again mourning the loss even more acutely as Justina and Viktor had been physically reunited after months of socially distant meet ups and video chat-based movie dates.

Thus, September found Viktor and I at loggerheads again and again, fighting about Justina or my perceptions of the situation or simply my unhappiness. I was triggered by so many things and began to harbor my own anger and resentment.

During those months, the threat had been temporarily removed, but their spending the full Labor Day Weekend together and then making plans for future holiday weekend dates had me tied up in knots, thrust back on that rollercoaster of deep, dark, dangerous emotions. I was severely struggling to stay sane as suicidal thoughts once again flooded my mind.

After the initial pain of Fall 2019, I had felt the guilt of cutting things off when Viktor had just gotten started and had promised him that he and Justina could have six months together. That half year came and went and here we were a year older, but perhaps no wiser on how best to move forward.

I felt him slipping away as his attention and interest in me waned, instead transferred from me to Justina and others. He no longer sought to explore sexual activities with me; he would forget to use my love language; he didn't capture our experiences in photos as he did with the others. All cues that left me feeling abandoned and bereft; I felt as if I was being replaced in pieces over time.

Yet for me, it had been about so much more than jealousy and while I tried to express my pain and suffering with Viktor, I felt that, at least initially, he didn't truly understand or get the immensity of what I was feeling. We talked, fought, made up and moved on and everything was fine for a while...Until it wasn't. Each time I found myself in a dark place; there was fear of loss, jealousy, envy, and a real quandary as to who I was anymore.

We had one more brief respite in early October as we celebrated my 50th birthday and then our 24th wedding anniversary. But we were soon back to the angst and anxiety.

The squeaky wheel gets the grease

In mid-October, I spent the weekend with my sister in Virginia, while Viktor spent the full weekend with Justina. It was already an emotionally tough situation for me due to the length of time he would be with her, some challenges that had occurred with scheduling and the anxiety I felt in anticipating time with my sister. Then, figuring out when we would be able to connect with one another during our absence became a challenge as well, adding to my torment.

While I was happy to see my sister, I was angry that the timing was foisted upon me and I was upset at the way my requests for contact during our absence from one another were received.

I wanted to talk to Viktor before bed, but he resisted because he didn't want to have to interrupt his plans with Justina to do so. Rather, he wanted to connect in the early evening instead. I bristled, but tried to accept what he was offering, yet I felt like I wasn't being seen or heard.

Coincidentally, during my visit, my sister and I listened to a podcast[15] featuring Jessica Fern, author of *PolySecure* and it was as if she were speaking directly to me. Yes, it was suddenly, abundantly clear that my anxious/preoccupied attachment style was at the heart of my pain and suffering regarding our open relationship. Was there jealousy? Yes, but jealousy was only one piece of this vast puzzle. It was my abandonment trauma (still not fully resolved), my insecure attachment style, a lack of self-love and yes, some jealousy and envy, all conspiring against me in this situation. It was clear to me that my insecurity was the real culprit, and I knew that it would not be an easy fix to overcome such a deep-seated mindset.

I spent a nearly sleepless night mulling things over and then returned to New York on Monday afternoon, ready to confront Viktor with my new-found revelations. After months of suffering, I had finally made the firm decision to put myself first, finding self-love and prioritizing my happiness and well-being. I was making myself a priority for perhaps the first time.

It was scary, but, once home, I told Viktor that I was choosing me. While the upshot was that it was monogamy or polyamory, I wanted him to determine what he truly needed. But I knew what was best for my mental health and emotional state; I needed the stability and security of monogamy...at least for now.

We tried to proceed with a few more weeks of the status quo, but it was still more than I could handle; I needed things to end. After many tear-filled conversations, we agreed to part ways with our other partners. Viktor spoke with Justina and I had a very jumbled conversation with Alex, breaking up with him for the sake of my sanity and for the sake of our marriage.

Yes, it was painful and dramatic, and I felt like shit, but I knew in my heart of hearts that it was the right decision for me and for our marriage — if we were to save our marriage. Frankly, at that point we

---

[15] Chambliss, Kitty. Jessica Fern Interview. *Loving Without Boundaries podcast.* October 3, 2020.

weren't sure it could be saved, but we knew that we had to put in the time and effort and really try before walking away from one another.

Those first few days were rough for both of us having cut off all contact with Justina and Alex. As we joked, it was an elimination diet as we went through the symptoms of withdrawal.

There was tremendous guilt at the hurt I had caused, feeling some overblown sense of responsibility. And, of course, there was the loss of our connection and communication.

Not surprisingly, it was a fragile time for us as a couple, as we navigated our break-ups and still had so much work to do to move our marriage forward. It was daunting as we wondered if we were headed toward divorce; something neither of us wanted, but both of us felt was a possibility.

Yet, we were committed to doing what was necessary to make things work or rather to repair and strengthen our bond. We continued to fight, but fortunately we began to find the skills to successfully de-escalate these conflicts, taking the lessons learned from each altercation to move forward instead of backward.

By early December, we had found our footing and, while we knew there was still much work to do, we felt that we had turned a corner and that divorce no longer loomed large. We breathed a collective sigh of relief, knowing that the worst was behind us. Moreover, I was keenly aware that I had my own internal demons and began to work with an individual therapist as well.

And, as Christmas and New Year's Eve rolled around, the security and surety of our relationship was fully restored. We recognized where we had gone astray and, while his relationship with Justina had been an issue, we admitted that our problems had started before they ever had met.

We had failed to fully cultivate and nurture our emotional intimacy, which we were now able to see, understand and take steps to correct. Viktor also had an interesting epiphany, noting that Justina was the first person to love him in his new incarnation after a big personal growth spurt. He apologized for not taking me along on his journey and this revelation further helped us heal.

As I worked with my therapist to address my various issues, I focused on setting clear boundaries; overcoming sexual trauma; healing from abandonment trauma; becoming more secure in my attachments; finding self-love and self-compassion; and learning where these early hurts stemmed from and how to move past them.

In addition to our weekly sessions, I was reading relevant books, completing workbooks, taking related classes and investing in better self-care. It almost began to feel like a full-time job, but I knew it was worth the time and energy.

On the same page

In a further effort to overcome my demons, I started to explore the use of psychedelics to do shadow work. Once on this path, I gave myself over to the process and was open to what would happen. As I took a medicinal dose of psilocybin, I had an emotionally, mentally and physically exhausting, four-hour trip, which was also extremely profound and productive. I learned so much from the experience and then began the process of slowly integrating those teachings, taking advantage of the window of neuroplasticity in which to make important and necessary cognitive changes.

In the wake of that experience, I felt better and stronger. During the trip, Viktor and I had an incredible moment as I felt the intensity of our love — spiritually, emotionally and physically — throughout my body, in every fiber of my being. It reinforced my belief that I was unable to give this all-encompassing type of love to anyone else. And further renewed my unwavering certainty that we truly were soulmates.

As we talked through these feelings and emotions, I felt as if he had returned to me after having been away for a long time. It was a final restoration of our marital bond. Yet, while I knew in my heart that he was mine, I also knew that I didn't own him. I needed to be able to let go and trust; to trust in our unconditional love that he would always come back to me. In many ways, he belonged to me, but he was not mine to possess.

Coincident with this work, we wrote up an extensive relationship agreement that outlined how we wanted to conduct ourselves in the context of our marriage. We ascertained our individual needs; set guidelines for honesty, communication and how to handle conflicts; and addressed how we wished to approach intimacy, emotional growth, self-care and the balance between dependence and independence. It felt wonderful to talk through these things, confirm our shared values and determine how we wished to live together as primary partners.

With this agreement firmly in place, we then turned our attention to an Appendix, which focused on our desires, boundaries, rules, etc. for being open. We clearly defined the ways in which our marriage would be monogamous (i.e., structural) and how it would be consensually non-monogamous. We delineated the hierarchical nature of our relationship and created our own scale of connection types, which ranged from Stranger to Soulmate.

We also addressed important issues such as one's energy and capacity to pursue external connections; how to manage scheduling; dealing with possible concerns regarding potential or new connections; spelling out permitted (and non-permitted) activities and being extremely specific with regard to safer sex practices. We ended with a list of hard limits, emotional support and safety guidelines.

Once this comprehensive document was completed, I gave Viktor the green light to see his FWB in late January. By this point, I was back in touch with Alex and was hopeful that he would consider resuming a romantic connection with me as I realized that I still had a lot to learn from him and that connection. Until he made his decision, we were simply friends and, while I admittedly hungered for more, I was grateful for his friendship. Viktor and I were technically back in an open marriage once again, but we hoped with more intention, clarity and guardrails this time around. In some ways we had come full circle and in others, it was the start of something exciting and new.

Epilogue

When we first opened up our marriage, I never considered the possibility of either of us falling in love. I know that to many this might seem preposterous (if not simply naïve), but I had a very narrow view of love. To me, love fell into three different, and distinct, categories: *familial love* (love for parents, siblings, children and other family connections); *friendship love* (I will watch your cat for you when you travel even though I don't really like cats) and *romantic love* (the all-consuming, heart, body, mind and soulmate love that I have for Viktor).

Consequently, when Viktor first told me that he was in love with Justina, I was devastated because I couldn't understand how his love for her fit into one of my categories without eclipsing his love for me. This obviously wasn't familial love; they were having sex so it went far beyond friendship love; so, it must be romantic love and thus, a replacement for the love he had for me. I tried to wrap my head around it and to make sense of how these two things could co-exist simultaneously: Viktor's love for Justina and Viktor's love for Jeannie. I repeatedly failed and it continued to eat at me, causing significant pain, confusion and loss.

More recently, as Viktor and I spent significant time talking about all that had happened between us as well as between him and Justina, I was starting to expand my view of love. I realized that due to abandonment trauma, insecure attachment and the lack of unconditional love from my mother, I had been closed off to love in many ways due to fear, distrust and a lack of self-worth. As I invested the time to heal and do the work, I was slowly trying to open my heart and mind to love.

Part of the work that Viktor and I were doing centered around the need for a shared vocabulary. We desperately wanted to be able to clearly communicate with one another and have the other fully understand what we meant by our words. This desire to create what I jokingly referred to as our "Family Dictionary," had been particularly challenging when it came to defining "love."

In this regard, love was such a tricky word. We use it all the time. I love ice cream; I love that sweater on you; I love the feel of the sun on my skin. And, when we interact on social media, we "heart" posts, photos and comments, distilling this four-letter word into an inconsequential signifier. Yet, on the other hand, we recognize that it is an extremely big deal when someone first says, "I love you," to you.

So where did that leave us? Confused? Maybe. At a minimum, we had been at a loss to truly distinguish what we meant by love, especially in a romantic context. Viktor and I had no doubt that we were soulmates and that our love was unique and special, but when he used the same word in connection with both Justina and me, he had been unable to clearly communicate the difference.

With this experience in mind, when I first started dating Alex, I began to think about the "L" word from my perspective. But I also knew that, unlike Viktor, I did not easily love or fall in love. In fact, I was fairly confident that I was not capable of loving more than one person at a time. Moreover, I worried that if I were to let myself be fully open to this possibility, it would significantly jeopardize our marriage (and possibly my mental health). To that end, I had remained hyper diligent about how much I let myself feel with Alex, carefully resisting the initial pull of New Relationship Energy, despite my declaration that I was letting go and staying open to possibility.

And yet, after we had broken up, I felt somewhat bereft at the loss of that relationship. I missed him; I missed us; and I wondered if, in fact, I had loved him to some degree. Not the type of love that I shared with Viktor, but some other, equally lovely, yet less intense, type of romantic love. I sought in vain to find the right word(s) to describe it. The closest I came was LOKE, but admittedly, although it did reflect the hierarchy I wished to denote, I found this word (an amalgamation of **LO**ve + li**KE**) to be a bit too flip.

From the very beginning of my relationship with Alex, I was unable to define things; it was so different from any previous relationship I had encountered during our open marriage. At that time, I had made the decision to let go of labels and simply enjoy what was, but now that these unidentified emotions still lingered, I felt called once again to make sense of them. Part of it was to understand what feelings I was capable of and part of it was to have a better sense of things going forward. More specifically, if what I felt for Alex *was* some type of love, then I could more easily understand and accept that Viktor's love for someone else (if similar in intensity to what I had with Alex) was *not* a threat or danger to our marriage.

In the aftermath of our respective break-ups, Viktor and I focused on repairing and strengthening our own relationship and love. We put in the time and effort to reconnect and to restore what had been lost. Yet, we found ourselves struggling to make meaning and to parse out different types of love. For a long time, it was a moving target, but as we worked tirelessly on our Relationship Agreement and then, later, on the Appendix, we started to somehow find a way to designate and differentiate among various emotional options more easily.

Are there 50 shades of love? I don't know, but I concede that there are certainly more nuances than the three I first described, and I am committed to being more open to love in its many guises.

Equally important, the work I have done on healing myself has been invaluable. While I wish it hadn't taken all of the heartache and anguish that it did to uncover all of my trauma, I am grateful to be on a (likely lifelong) healing path. I feel that I have made significant progress in a few short months and have learned so much about myself.

During this time, I read a beautiful book, *Come As You Are*, by Emily Nagoski, a resource I wished had been around back in the mid-to-late 1990s when I first dealt with my lack of desire. Her words and knowledge have been incredibly uplifting, enlightening and encouraging as I have continued to focus on my sexual awakening.

Of course, that's what this journey was initially all about; a way for me to get my groove back. But it has been so much more, more than I could have imagined; perhaps more than I bargained for. But it has been my destiny to find my desire, heal my heart and truly awaken my authentic self.

Recommended Reading

Castellanos, Madeleine. *Wanting to Want: What Kills Your Sex Life and How to Keep It Alive.* New York: 2014.

Nagoski, Emily. *Come as You Are: The Surprising New Science that Will Transform Your Sex Life.* New York: Simon Schuster, 2015.

Ryan, Christopher and Jethá, Cacilda. *Sex at Dawn.* New York: HarperCollins, 2010.

Taormino, Tristan. *Opening Up: A Guide to Creating and Sustaining Open Relationships.* Minneapolis: Cleis Press, 2008.

Thomashauer, Regena. *Mama Gena's School of Womanly Arts: Using the Power of Pleasure to Have Your Way with the World.* New York: Simon Schuster, 2003.

Thomashauer, Regena. *Pussy: A Reclamation.* Carlsbad: Hay House, Inc., 2016.

Urbaniak, Kasia. *Unbound: A Woman's Guide To Power.* London: Vermilion, 2020.

Winston, Sheri. *Anatomy of Female Arousal: Secret Maps to Buried Pleasure.* Kingston: Mango Garden Press, 2011.